Cover design by Stephen J. Catizone, 2014

1st Edition Printing - 2014
2nd Edition Printing – 2016

Edited by Edin Crowe – 2016

Printed in the U.S.A.
Createspace

The information herein is not intended to diagnose, treat, or cure, and should not be taken in place of medical advice by a licensed, medical physician.

ISBN – 13:978-1540424303
ISBN – 10:1540424308

A Semicolon Kind of Life;

Living & Healing With Colorectal Cancer

Krista D'Ambroso

For Jackie McGrath, PA,
thank you for saving my life!
To my grandmother, Alice
Daniel Pritchard, who always
believed in my writing, and kept
every scrap of paper I ever wrote on
to prove it.

I also dedicate this book to everyone who's
trying to figure things out with their health,
whether it's with cancer, or some other
health issue, and of course to the millions of
people
who have lost their lives prematurely to disease.

TABLE OF CONTENTS

Acknowledgements

In starting off, I would like to add my thanks to everyone who's been a part of this book. First, my great appreciation to the very talented graphic artist, Steven James Catizone for the beautiful cover art he designed for me. I hope we can work together on my future projects.

Next, I would like to thank Jackie McGrath, PA. She was the first person (after two horribly symptomatic years) who took my symptoms seriously, and gave me the tools I needed to get me to the next step in my healing. To me, Jackie is the person who really saved my life.

To my friends and family who supported me through the good times and bad; by visiting me in the hospital, taking me to doctor's appointments and treatments, and for their overall love and support. Couldn't have done much without you guys; especially my Mother, Karen, who continues to take me to my appointments to this day.

To David, for all the hours of waiting and waiting, and waiting some more, and all the driving, driving, and driving some more. You were my rock when I needed you!

To my online family and support of people who are still in the healing phases of cancer, and to those I care about who died as a result of this very unbiased disease. You gave me the inspiration to figure it out, and aided in my belief that I could.

To my readers; may you find the good health you deserve. It's my greatest wish that my journey will help you on yours.

Thank you.

INTRODUCTION

I was born a poor white child in a semi-ghetto region of Southern California...

Now that we have THAT out of the way, let's talk about CANCER!

Yes, that's right...I said it! I said, "Let's talk about CANCER!" Without fear, without hesitation, and without a single worry that the word might choke me to death while it crept up my throat, I said it! Believe it, or not, my fingers didn't fall off as I typed it, either. I mean, heck, I summed up my childhood in one single sentence, so the most important aspect of my life must be happening right now, at this very moment; writing to discuss one of the scariest topics in the world today; about a disease that takes thousands of lives every year, and leaves those who survive it with debilitating after-affects. You're reading me right now, either cradling me gently in your hands, or straining to see my words against the bright light of an electronic devise, possibly because it's a topic you're familiar with because someone you know or love has it. Maybe you're just curious about the subject matter. Perhaps you're enthusiastic about different types of health regimes. There's an even better chance that you're one of the many cancer recipients dangling precariously at the end of your chemo rope without a safety net or glass of water to catch you when you fall. Well, whichever boat you're rowing, you're here, so let's get thriving!

What a beautiful start to a magical journey; I mean

knowing right off the starting line that you can come out of this ahead.

And that's exactly what this is going to be; a magical journey that proves you can come out ahead!

If I had to sum up the contents of this book in one paragraph, here is what the advertisement might read:

"Calling all cancer adventurers, journeymen, laymen, and expert travelers...The ship called "Cancer" is setting sail, and all are invited to disembark, now! Say "Thank You" to cancer for its array of entertaining, if not painful show stopping productions, then graciously move on to better and brighter things. Such as LIVING! Send that ship on its way as a ghost ship, never to see landfall again."

Inside these pages there are not a lot of documented studies telling us our odds of dying from colorectal cancer. No gimmicks on how mixing one part baking soda to three parts cottage cheese will work wonders on killing it. No promises that any one program or system will cure all, or any disease.

This is the story of how I'm defeating one of the deadliest cancers on the planet without chemotherapy, simply by developing my own system for doing so. By dealing with my cancer on MY terms, and how other people can benefit from what I've learned. Above all, it's my hope that this story, my story, can, and will motivate and inspire ANYONE on the journey to a healthier, happier self, achieve it. The information in this book can be useful to anyone, not just those with colorectal cancer. Colorectal cancer just happens to be my disease. My personal formula is meant to give ideas for someone else in developing their own, personal healing program.

To me, CANCER is kind of like a self-deprecating disease. It's our own bodies turning on themselves and wreaking havoc among our healthy cells; our cells mutating and transforming into something other than what they were originally meant to be, and then spreading their malignancy to every other cell in the Universe that is our body.

In my own research over the past decade, I've come across a lot of scientific data to both support, and debunk the theories of what exactly cancer is, and how to treat it. Most importantly, I've met people with real experiences that told me more about what I needed to know than any twenty studies ever could. It's the real experiences that teach us and better separate the truth from theory. Let's just face it; science isn't a perfect science.

I'm not here to tell anyone not to do something, or to definitely do something else to treat their CANCER or disease.

Don't worry, I'm not going to capitalize the word CANCER during the entire book! I just want to signify the tremendous power that word has. It invokes a particularly strong feeling in people when they both hear, and say it, and it usually isn't a positive one. Let me try to change that, if you don't mind.

Here's how I take some of the negative power out of the word CANCER. The first half of that word gives ME the power. It is "CAN". The other half of the word can stand for Conditioned Emotional Response, or C.E.R.. I CAN beat my CANCER by changing my CONDITIONED EMOTIONAL RESPONSES to it. CAN

C.E.R. The word has a different kind of power to it for me now...a positive one. Positivity is the only cure for negativity and in changing my response to that word to a positive one, the word no longer invokes a bad feeling when I hear, see, or taste it.

My story may not be the most incredible cancer survival story ever told, but it's definitely a relative one. Other individuals have learned how to beat or control their illness by similar methods, some of which I will discuss, as well as other suggestions pertaining to what I am doing through experimentation, and trial and error.

I've tried to include every aspect of what I've done, and elaborated on the aspects that I thought were most important in my survival. I don't consider myself any great philosopher, and I'm not a psychology expert by any means, but in my studies, I have been fortunate to gain enough insight into the human psyche to enable myself to achieve the attitude and behaviors that were imperative to my healing. They are practice makes perfect tasks that anyone can do without needing a ton of money or special expertise to do.

I have included resources in the appendix for my fellow cancerians on where to find financial assistance, alternative therapies, relevant books and articles, and other useful information to aid anyone in permanently disembarking that cancer ship once and for all.

In closing this introduction, I just want to say, it is my strongest belief that all of us CAN manage, and even CURE ourselves of just about anything. Of course we can! We're alive, so we're already survivors, now it's time to become THRIVER survivors and say adios, adieu, and auf wiedersehen to our diseases.

The Nastiest Little Fairy

I always know when she is near,
by the urgent burning in my rear.

She shows up when I'm having fun,
to fill my bowels like a loaded gun.

The painful cramping starts 'bout then,
hot lava churning from within.

Subtle she can never be,
are those gaseous sounds coming out of me?

I reason with her every day,
"witch just stay the ~BLEEP~ away!"

She has a sense of humor at least,
she comes when the toilet's farthest to reach.

I'm usually quite the gentle soul,
but if I ever got hold of her, I just don't know!

First, I'd see her point of view,
having to be the fairy of poo.

I imagine she is cruelly teased,
by the fairies whose jobs are to flower the trees.

They call her mean and horrible names,
and don't let her join in their fairytale games.

Maybe she sits in a corner alone,
blubbering tears like a mad little crone.

Then she releases her anger on me,
twisting my bowels from point-A, to point-B.

For a moment my tears and pity are for her,
then very quickly that moment is over.

I hate to admit it, but I've only one wish,
that someday that fairy becomes fairy dust
squish!

1.
SYMPTOMATIC CHAOS

I started noticing subtle changes in my body at the time of my separation from my husband in 2004. I was 35 years old, and working a temporary job at a major department store. I first noticed that a salad I had eaten the day before, exited my body pretty much the same as it had entered; whole and undigested. I had been under a lot of stress having to cohabitate with my husband after a year-long separation as we tried to negotiate a divorce. My job didn't offer health insurance, so I went to the clinic for advice. The doctor there told me that what I was experiencing wasn't all that unusual, but he recommended I see a GI doctor, anyway. All fine and good, but without health insurance, that wasn't happening.

Not long after that, I got an abscessed cyst in the middle of my chest that had to be excised there in the clinic. The doctor wasn't able to anesthetize the area very well, so I was unable to endure the entire surgery. As a result, only half of the cyst sac was removed, leaving a gaping wound that had to heal open. It took a long time to heal, and kept getting infected.

Six months later, I was able to move from the marital house into an apartment of my own in another town with a new job, just days before my ex-husband was to move his new girlfriend in. The divorce had been a drawn out nightmare, and my new job was even more stressful than my last. I started noticing blood in my stool sometime within the next few months, but didn't think much of it. I wasn't even positive it was blood, or so I kept telling myself.

I got a better paying job the next year doing the exact same thing (working with brain injured adults). It was a commute, and more emotionally stressful than my last job.

Within three days of starting the new job, I was bowled over in the bathroom with the most horrible abdominal cramps I'd ever had. When I was finally able to leave the bathroom, my supervisor gave me a couple of pain pills, and a fellow employee drove me to the emergency room.

After sitting in the ER for several hours, the pain subsided. They CT scanned me, and did an ultra sound. What they found was a huge gallstone. They didn't seem concerned about the rectal bleeding and mucous I told them occasionally happened. They said the pain was from the gallstone, and sent me home with a referral to a GI doctor.

I knew I was going to have to get my gallbladder removed as soon as possible, but I would have to wait at least three months at the new job before I qualified for health insurance.

I was almost to that three month mark when the abdominal pains became unbearable. Another trip to the ER, and again, nothing found but the gallstone. I had become downed with infection after infection over the next few weeks. The doctors thought it was a real bad sinus infection, and then decided that wasn't it. They finally admitted they didn't know what was causing it.

15

The antibiotics weren't working, and I was losing a lot of time at work. Not good for only being there a couple of months. While all of this was going on, a political situation at work was getting uglier and uglier until it boiled to a head one night.

A supervisor had put in a complaint about me and one of the other supervisors. Apparently we were taking too long on a project, and he thought we were goofing off. The head manager called all three of us in one night and we were interrogated like the Spanish Inquisition. A shouting match ensued, with accusations of racism and favoritism flying around the room. I sat in my seat and cried; the whole time expecting violence to erupt at any moment. At least that's how it felt at the time. I'll never know for sure what exactly was going on with all of that, but it was the least of my problems. I was so sick the next day I was out of work for the next two weeks, and not getting any better. I quit the job, and spent nearly a month in bed. I couldn't afford to go to the clinic anymore, and felt it never helped for very long anyway. Whatever it was, it was going to have to run its course.

I was a month unemployed, going back and forth between looking for work, and being too ill with infections and fevers to get out of bed.

I found a job cleaning houses that was extremely hard on my body, but was usually only about three to five hours of work per day. It kept me afloat, and eventually the infections got better. Energy drinks triggered horrible bathroom issues, but they kept my energy level up well enough to work the short, but labor intensive days.

At the end of 2005, I became involved with a nice man named David and fell into a whirlwind romance with him.

16

We moved out of my apartment a few months later to a nice little farm on the outskirts of town where we got lowered rent in exchange for taking care of the animals on the property.

There were llamas, miniature horses, donkeys, chickens, a beautiful black swan, an emu, a miniature cow, and several other animals. Being the animal lover that I am, I was in paradise and happy for the first time in many years. I had always promised my miniature schnauzer, Pebbles, that someday we would live on a farm (she loved horses, and could sit and stare at them for hours), and now, in her 11th year of life, we were living the dream! Happiness abounded...

But time was running out for me.

I had taken on another job on the weekends as a relief for the house manager at a residential psychiatric facility. It supplemented my income just enough. It was a 12 hour on, 12 hour off, shift, Friday and Saturday nights. The clients were mostly easy to deal with, but I had problems with one of the younger clients who was completely non-compliant and had me calling the police on him regularly. I found myself having to make hard decisions on how to handle him every weekend, and it put me in a perpetual state of stress my body was incapable of handling. I was finally learning that my propensity for dealing with stress was low, and that it was my body that would suffer the consequences of it more than my mentality.

It wasn't long before I was getting severely sick with bathroom issues both at the job, and at home. So much blood was leaving my body through my rectum, I felt physically exerted from it. I could tell I was colon blocked. Barely any stool would come out most of the time, and sometimes I would have to vomit because I just wasn't able to pass anything the other way. I spent a lot of time having to clean up my messes in the bathroom at work after the clients had all gone to bed. Luckily, since the job was at night, I had some privacy. Night time was becoming the most usual time my body would act out; while trying to relax.

The pain was becoming excruciating. I was fearful of food, but whether I ate or not, blood kept coming out in puddles. I mixed my time between being bowel incontinent, and going to the bathroom thirty times per day.

My housekeeping job was suffering badly. I wasn't able to clean as fast as my teammates, and spent way too much time in the bathroom at client's houses bleeding out. I drank energy drinks constantly and they made the bathroom issues much worse. They were the only thing making it possible for me to keep working during the day.

I began having problems with my co-workers at my housekeeping job. I'm a very easy person to get along with, but my attitude and motivation was at an all-time low. I was even having major conflicts with my boss, and challenged her on everything. Looking back, I know it was from exhaustion and constant irritability. It didn't matter where I was, home, or otherwise. I was uncomfortable everywhere.

By April of 2007, I could no longer handle the physicality of cleaning houses, and had to quit. I held onto the psychiatry job, even though going there was a nightmare, and I often wondered when my shifts came up, if I could make the drive to the facility, pick up the clients and take them to the other house before I had a bathroom emergency.

I started a little online business so I could work at home selling women's clothing that helped us out a bit, but David was working full time, AND doing almost all of the work with the farm animals. I had three cats, two dogs, and a bearded dragon that also took David's energy. Things were getting harder for both of us. I was still able to pay my part of the rent, but nothing else.

I began thinking I was going to die. In fact, I wished every day that I would die.

I began having fantasies about an isolated island with a beautiful blue lagoon that had a long pier in it. There was a gazebo at the end that had long, sheer curtains hanging off the eaves. Inside the gazebo was a comfy bed, a television set, and tons of yummy food I could imagine eating. My favorite cat, Mouser, who passed away in 1998 was always laying on the bed waiting for me.

In this other realm, I was free of pain and only peace and tranquility existed there. I began to believe this place was real and each night in bed, I would go there and pray that the next time I woke up, that's where I would really be. Dying was the only thing I looked forward to anymore, but strangely, it was one of the things that actually kept me going. Just imagining the place took me out of my suffering for at least a little while.

One of the other things that helped during this time was my big ragdoll cat, Malachi. He would come onto the bed and lay the full length of his body on my tummy at night. The pressure of his weight would bring me some relief. He never used to do this before I got sick, and he has never done it since.

The bathroom issues had gotten to the point that in

order to produce a bowel movement at all, I had to soak in a hot bath for however long it would take to liquefy the stool, and then trying to pass it was an act of torture.

On better days, I wouldn't leave the house unless I was wearing a diaper and I had to know exactly where the bathroom was wherever we were going. If it was a "one stall" bathroom, and someone was in it, I would have to use the men's, which was embarrassing when I got caught.

Life had completely lost its color for me. I just wished it would end.

Another ER visit and CT scan in June revealed nothing, even though I told the doctor I was bleeding to death. Yes, she agreed I was anemic to the point of ALMOST needing a blood transfusion. So she wrote a recommendation for iron supplements, and drugged me up so badly, David had to drag me out of the ER. They gave me another GI referral, too.

I knew it was cancer.

I knew I was dying a very slow, painful death, but I believed there was NOTHING I could do about it. If the ER and clinic wouldn't help me, who would?

People who knew me told me it couldn't be cancer. Even the doctor's at the clinic said I was too young. Too young...I wondered if that was even possible. Didn't little children get cancer? I was 38. Really? Too young?

I made one more attempt at the clinic.

A physician's assistant named Jackie, took one look at me and my family history, and wanted to know why I hadn't had a colonoscopy yesterday. When I told her my story, she told me about a program called CMS designed for people in the county experiencing a medical emergency who did not have insurance. She told me where to go, and how to apply for it.

After a few issues with the CMS program messing up my name, I had a GI appointment scheduled a month later, on July 31st.

A ray of hope cleared the clouds! If jumping up and down wouldn't have felt like my bowels were going to fall out, I would've done it, for sure!

I prepared for the consultation by documenting a 24 hour period of my life. I described each bathroom visit, and what occurred therein.

When I looked at the paper on the way to see the doctor the next day, I was amazed at how I'd been living for so long and how the progression had come to what it was. Potty visits every 10-30 minutes, blood and mucus filling the toilet, debilitating abdominal cramps, off and on vomiting...I prayed the GI doctor could help me.

He was the kindest doctor I had met up to that point. After dealing with only ER doctors who were totally apathetic to my situation, this sweet and gentle doctor was a very pleasant change.

His name was Brad Moore. A youngish doctor, probably younger than me, who might have been a military doctor before joining UCSD. He had a slight Southern accent we thought might have been Arkansasian, or Tennessian, like all the relatives on my Mother's side of the family had. There was a lot of comfort in that familiar accent.

He listened to my story, taking notes the whole time with very few questions. Upon finishing, I told him my fear was that it was cancer. He said it wasn't likely because I was too young. This disheartened me.

21

It had to be cancer.

My greatest fear in the world at that point was that they wouldn't be able to find what was wrong with me, at all. They hadn't so far, with the exception of a gallstone I KNEW wasn't causing all of the problems I was having, and since everyone thought I was too young to have colon cancer, I was sure they wouldn't find the problem. At this time, I hadn't lost my faith in doctors and wasn't as self-assertive as I learned to be later. I insisted on trusting they knew what they were doing. It was a complete mystery to me why they hadn't found out what my problem was just from my symptoms, if they knew anything at all.

My condition had taken two years to deteriorate to the place it currently was, and had worsened exponentially within the last few months.

Yes, I hoped it was cancer. I figured they could at least treat that, and I would at long last have some relief from all the pain and suffering I was in. I wasn't thinking of any other consequences at that time. I didn't care about consequences. The worst consequence was death, and I was more than prepared for that!

Regardless of Dr. Moore's belief that my problem was not cancer related, he scheduled the colonoscopy for two days later.

Now anyone who has done the preparation for a colonoscopy knows it's quite the experience. Not everyone has the same reaction to the poop juice (golytly/halflytly) that has to be consumed to clean the bowels out, but as prepared as I was (diapers, keeping close to the bathroom, etc.), there are no words that can accurately describe the experience. I highly recommend it. There isn't much that can build a person's character better

22

than a bowel prep, especially if there are other people around.

For me, the diapers were useless. It was unfortunate that I didn't figure that out until afterwards.

I had been told that the poop juice would start working within 15 minutes to an hour after beginning the drink. After four hours, and the poop juice nearly gone, it still hadn't kicked in. I was beginning to think it wasn't going to work for me at all!

Just as that thought had entered my mind, I was literally in the bathroom from 8 pm that night, until 6 am the following morning when we had to start getting ready to leave. If I stepped out of the bathroom for just a minute, like I did ONE time...well, let's just leave it at that. Cleaned out...Amen!

The rest of the morning at the GI's was very tense for both David and I. I could feel his nervousness. For me, it was a huge relief to not have to go to the bathroom every ten minutes. However, my body didn't really know that, and was still giving me the feelings like I needed to go.

The colonoscopy was scheduled for 10 am, but they didn't get me into the procedure room until almost 11. By then I was a jumble of nerves. I wondered if it was really going to happen after all.

There were three people ahead of me; obviously I was a squeeze in, for that, and for many other reasons, I would be forever grateful to Dr. Moore.

One by one the patients got wheeled away until finally it was my turn.

The procedure room was not warm and inviting, but Dr. Moore and his nurses, were. I was talkative until they started the IV drugs.

My body immediately went all warm and fuzzy with the Demerol and versed drugs entering my system. It was a great feeling. It reminded me of the time in the ER when they drugged me up so badly I couldn't see straight. Not a bad feeling at all. In fact, it was a feeling I would spend the next half decade looking forward to because it was the only time in my existence I was completely out of pain.

I was lying on my left side with a TV monitor directly in front of me. Actually, the monitor was in front of him, and he was behind me.

I could see the scope entering my body, and was stunned that everything was so magnified.

My colon looked smooth and pink on the monitor, moving and breathing on its own, even though the scope was probably the only thing actually moving. Every once in a while a fast moving river of neon green liquid would rush passed the camera. I had no idea at the time that it was bile, because the fluid looked unnaturally green. Probably a result of the TV monitor's color settings.

Soon, the TV screen seemed to darken, and the walls of the colon narrowed. The pink walls turned dark-red and swollen. Eventually the circular tunnel was nearly devoid of an opening and the flesh became twisted and malformed, heaving, and oozing blood in various places along its mass. Even though I knew what I was looking at; it was a hideously gnarled tumor, my mind was not at all impressed. I can understand how people get addicted to those pain drugs! I knew what I was looking at, but I simply didn't care. I remember thinking, "huh, that's really ugly", then I shrugged it off, and continued watching as a little three-pronged, metal arm came out of nowhere and plucked a huge chunk of flesh off the

24

monstrosity. It then retracted in, and the camera squeezed on passed the tumor. I remember thinking, "that didn't hurt. I think that should've hurt?"

I saw the little metal arm come out again one or two more times after passing the mass to pluck off some more raised tissues, then my memory faded.

My next memory was waking up to see the three patients who had gone in before me in three, little, curtained alcoves. They were all in various stages of getting ready to leave. My gurney was against the wall across from them, segregated by myself.

I saw a nurse walk by. She glanced at me and the look she had on her face was a look I wouldn't see the last of. I can only describe it as a look of great pity, but it's really a more complicated look than that. I guess I can go a bit further and be truly honest about what the look invokes. It says, "I'm looking at a dead person, and I feel so horrible for them. I'd better smile."

I drifted back to sleep.

I don't know how much time passed before I was awake again. This time, I sat myself up. Immediately Dr. Moore came into the room, and sat next to me on the bed. He put a hand on my knee, and he said very gently that he was sorry, but they found a mass.

I asked if it was malignant, and he said it was.

"What next?" I asked, still groggy.

"Probably chemo." He said.

"What stage is it?" I asked, not really understanding that he couldn't tell that from a colonoscopy.

He said he didn't know and more tests would have to be done. Then he asked me if I wanted him to tell David. I said I could do that.

25

I was dressed and sitting in a wheelchair when David came into the room. I told him it was cancer, and he just looked at the ground. During all this time of having to deal with my illness, I'm sure he knew just as well as I did that it was going to be cancer.

The doctor wanted blood taken and a CT scan done right away. I had no idea of the roller coaster ride we were about to embark on, but this was definitely the moment of take-off.

Before I had left the hospital that day, we had an appointment with the colorectal surgeon, an oncologist, and another CT scan scheduled, all within a week. Suddenly everything was hurried and rushed as if time were an issue, when I had been sick for years.

The mass was so large, it was causing an obstruction. Duh. It had been bleeding so much I needed a blood transfusion ASAP. Duh. The CT scan couldn't be read past my lower colon because the tumor was so large the contrast couldn't get passed it. Well duh. That last bit was a "DUH" moment I had while on the CT table immediately after diagnosis.

The tech came in and told me they were unable to scan the lower part of my pelvis. The contrast wasn't showing up there. It took me about five minutes of them running around trying to figure out what was wrong, and of me thinking, "hm", when it dawned on me that the contrast wasn't able to get past the tumor which had been blocking everything else trying to get passed this whole time!

Something else I hadn't known till that moment was that the tech's weren't given any information about why I was there, or what they were looking for. This seemed illogical and impractical to me. I made it a habit from then on to tell the tech's why I was getting scanned. It has helped when there were any questions as to why I needed contrast for one scan, and not another, and it has also solved blood work questions, and so on. It would've helped in this situation, tremendously.

So I was going to need an enema before this first CT scan could be done.

A doctor came in and gave me the enema right then and there on the scanning table. It was only the first humiliation in a long line of humiliations that would litter my life from that point on! Remember when I said there wasn't much else that builds character better than a bowel prep? Well, rectal exams, doctor induced enemas, and sitting on the toilet in front of a room full of people have the bowel prep beat by a long shot.

At any rate, the "DUH" moment solved the mystery as to why the CT scans done in the ER all those times never revealed the 3cm tumor wreaking havoc in my rectum. No one in the ER cared enough to figure out why the CT's weren't complete, and I can only imagine how many different people dropped the ball and maintained their silence on that one! You may be thinking major lawsuit? I'll talk about that in a minute.

As it was, the pompous little bastard was finally exposed in the bright, shimmering light of CT film. A star amongst the other two benign polyps they found, its identity no longer a mystery my body was trying so desperately and for so many years, to expose.

Oh, don't worry. I'm a lot calmer now than I was back then.

At the time, I was furious.

I was furious that I had been treated like garbage by the

healthcare establishment. I was furious that my cancer had been allowed to fester inside me, torturing me, and slowly killing me while the technology to help me was right there staring me in the face, yet not available to me. I was furious that I was denied proper life-saving treatments because of my income level and insurance status. I was furious that the system was set up to help people in my situation, but nobody cared enough to inform me about it, even though they could see I was in a lot of trouble. Not until I met Jackie, the one and only person throughout this whole experience who stepped up and held out her hand to me. She was the ONLY person in two years who gave me that very simplistic information that saved my life.

A lot of people in the healthcare field have helped me since Jackie, but if it wasn't for her, I never would've met any of them. I would've endured a lot more suffering, and eventually would have withered away and died.

It's the reason this book is dedicated to her, and if I can ever find her, I won't be able to thank her enough for that one simple act she did of doing her job.

I hope that one day all healthcare professionals will realize the true importance of their jobs and the impact they have on our society. It only takes one person to do one kind act to change the world, and healthcare providers are in the best position to do that.

I had decided in those early days that I was going to do something to change it in my own way as soon as I got better. There was no doubt in my mind that I wouldn't get better, and no doubt that I wouldn't make a change in the way things were done.

I knew I had a lawsuit against the hospital on many levels. Besides the patient dumping, we had found out that they switched one of my earlier CT scans with someone else's, giving me a false (inaccurate) diagnosis of a liver hemangioma that no one even told me about.

David and I pursued the lawsuit briefly until the attorney who was going to take our case told us we'd have to do all the footwork. She said there was a cap on the amount of money we would be granted, also. Though it wasn't about the money, at the time, we would have had to use a lot of our own money and the lawsuit could have been drawn out for years.

Although a lawsuit may have been a great way to bring about some much needed changes in patient care at that hospital, I was in absolutely no place to take on that responsibility. I already suspected that my cancer was stress induced, so I had to pick my battles carefully. There were so many things to consider, and all were time sensitive.

For one thing, the time to file the lawsuit had a six month window. I'd be right in the throes of my cancer treatments.

I made the decision to drop the idea of a lawsuit, even though I got two more chances to file later on.

For me, there were better ways to make changes in the world that didn't require a stress inducing lawsuit. Writing this book was one of them.

2.
AND WE'RE OFF!

David, my Mother, and I, met with the oncologist that Thursday. He was a jovial young doctor, fresh out of residency. He gave me a rectal exam and could feel the tumor with his finger. The ER doctors could feel the tumor, too, but they all assumed it was internal hemorrhoids.

We discussed the course of treatment I would do.

The tumor was too big to be removed without taking my entire rectum, so a course of chemo and radiation would have to be done first. The chemo, an old tried and true was called 5FU. I would do six weeks of continual dosing. That meant I would have a little contraption called a port-cath surgically implanted under the skin of my chest with an IV going into my jugular vein. The port-cath looked like a multi-tiered flying saucer, and was the diameter of a quarter. The chemo would be plugged into the port-cath via a little pump I had to carry around with me 24/7. It would be in an oversized fanny pack that fit the pump, the chemo bag, AND the excess tubing that connected everything to the port inside it. I couldn't get a clear picture from this description, and it really is something you'd have to visually see to make sense of.

Every week I would go to the infusion center to have the chemo bag refilled, and to get a 2-4 hour dose of the chemo, another substance called leucovorin, and a steroid drug (decadron) to prevent vomiting while in the infusion center.

I didn't understand how all of this would work while he was describing it to me, but I didn't like it. Of course I didn't like it. Who would? I was terrified of what all these substances would do to me in the long run. Did anyone even know?

The radiation would be done in either 25, or 30 zaps, every day except the weekends while I was on the chemo. It was their hope that the chemo and radiation done together would amplify the affects, and shrink the tumor.

One thing I really liked about the plan was the idea of shrinking the tumor. Being able to go to the bathroom again like a normal person was too tempting to say no to.

After the chemo radiation, the plan continued with a colon resection to rid my body of whatever was left of the tumor, and to remove fourteen lymph nodes in the area. Then I'd have to do some adjuvant chemo called FOLFOX for six months after the surgery to kill all the little loose floating cancer cells that might be present in my body. They referred to it as "mop-up" chemo. Before any of this was to start, I would have to get a blood transfusion.

The blood transfusion scared me more than anything else I had heard so far. On top of cancer, I was going to get AIDS! I actually didn't know all the different kinds of problems a blood transfusion could cause, but I was sure they were numerous. I didn't bother doing any research on the possible effects of a blood transfusion. Sometimes you just have to get it done. I was definitely feeling the urgency from everyone involved, as well as from the symptoms I was experiencing from the anemia.

I made the appointment to have the blood transfusion before we left the cancer center.

31

The radiation would be supervised by yet another doctor, so we made an appointment with her, too.

I met with the colorectal surgeon the following day.

Dr. R. was a small woman who looked several years younger than me, though she couldn't have been. She was very professional and pleasant, and seemed like she really knew what she was doing. She said she suspected that I was probably a stage III, and that there was a good chance the tumor had progressed through the fatty tissue and into my uterus. An MRI would have to be done before anything else. She also said she didn't think I would have to have a temporary colostomy, or poop bag as it's so called, attached to my side. That was a huge relief! Briefly, for those who don't know what a colostomy is, an incision is made on the side of the abdomen where a portion of the intestines comes out (a stoma), and a bag is glued to the body where the intestines can empty the poop into the bag. This diversion allows for the intestines to heal from a surgery. Some people have permanent colostomies because their colons have either been removed, or for some other reason why the intestines can't be used.

In the meanwhile, my suffering continued.

Everything was happening quickly, but it was all preparation, not treatment. I felt like opting out of shrinking the tumor and just having the rectum removed, but the prospect of having a permanent poop bag kept my decisions in check.

I got the MRI, my first one, and entered into yet another humiliation.

They needed to get a good picture of my uterus and believe it or not, they have a tool for that. Just imagine a dildo with ectoplasm all over it, and you get the picture.

This was also the first time someone had to access my port-cath.

I had had the port-cath surgically implanted a week earlier by two surfer-dude radiologists that each looked about 12. It was another conscious sedation type surgery that I was able to remember clearly, since the versed, once again, didn't work on me. Versed is the drug they give you for conscious sedation so you won't remember what happened to you during the procedure.

The port-cath procedure entailed a lot of jabbing, stabbing, and shoving to get the thing under the skin. It wasn't a fun procedure, though it didn't hurt, I felt the pressure of it. It itched, more than hurt, afterwards, and that never ended for the two years I had it.

So during the MRI, they not only had to put the ectoplasmic dildo in me, but they had to fill me with IV contrast, too. So the tech wanted to use the port-cath for the IV. Okay, I agree! Not getting poked over and over again in the arm sounded like a really good deal! It was as good a time as any to test the ole girl out, I thought. Unfortunately, they couldn't find any lidocaine to numb the port-cath area before putting in the special port-cath needle. "Okay", I say. "Is it going to hurt, or something?" "Naw," the tech says, "probably not." So I let them do it. I should've known after seeing the size of the needle that things weren't going to go so well. I never let anyone touch that sucker without lidocaine ever again, and there would be many times when nurses would want to. It was VERY painful, to say the least.

Thankfully, after all that, the tumor had not breached my uterus after all. That would have caused a whole other set of problems, and I really didn't need any more problems.

The blood transfusion was completed, and I was able to start my treatments the same day.

I met my radiation oncologist who was also very pleasant. I started the radiation the same day as the chemo.

Meanwhile, my poor, little, dog, Pebbles, had been having seizures over the past year, and we had finally stabilized her on barbiturates that seemed to prevent them.

A week after I started my treatments, Pebbles had a stroke and had to be put to sleep. I can't linger on this subject too long, but it was one of the worst days of my life. It put me into a state of hopelessness that's impossible to describe. Anyone who's lost a beloved companion animals understands. I missed her so much it made me sicker than the chemo.

I decided to get another little dog for my emotional health just a couple of weeks after Pebbles died.

The new puppy was a seven week old pug weighing no more than 3 lbs. We named her Rainbow and took her to all my appointments and treatments.

Every weekday David drove home from work forty minutes away to pick me and Rainbow up and drive another 45 minutes back down the hill into San Diego where my cancer center was for a ten minute radiation treatment, then 45 minutes back home again. The dedication he had was remarkable, and I'll always be thankful for what he did for me.

The treatments were rough, and I wasn't able to drive or do much of anything. I was tired all the time, and was still experiencing terrible bathroom issues. Nothing was getting any better after the first few weeks, and to add insult to injury, I was even more uncomfortable from the issues the treatments were causing.

I quit my psychiatric job not long after starting chemo. I couldn't concentrate well enough to do anything right, and it wasn't safe for me to drive. Even if it wasn't a job that required all my faculties, I still would've quit.

The house-manager nicknamed me Robo-Krista because of the weird gasping sounds the chemo pump made. I thought that was hilarious, and it lifted my spirits.

As much as I wanted to stay there (that horrible client that had caused me so much grief, had finally been gotten rid of), it wasn't the kind of job where mistakes could be blown off. I also knew that I had to greatly reduce the stress in my life if I was going to heal. I left the job with the intention of coming back when my treatments were finished.

While all of this was going on, Rainbow, our new pug puppy, was horribly sick. She was diagnosed with giardia first, then bordetella that turned into pneumonia. Back and forth doctor appointments for me, and back to back doctor appointments for Rainbow. It was a super challenging time.

Dr. R. had aged my tumor as being 3-5 years old. Right smack at the time my divorce had started.

All kinds of memories came flooding back about that whole experience, and I remembered a moment during my separation with my ex-husband when I just fell to pieces and snapped.

I thought I was having a nervous breakdown at the time. I had just gotten off the phone with my ex. We had been trying to get back together after being separated for six months. I heard a woman in the background on the phone, and when I asked him who it was, he told me it was his girlfriend. At that moment, I felt like my whole world had collapsed on itself. I knew for certain my fourteen year relationship was over. It was hard to breathe, and I couldn't move my legs for a good fifteen minutes. Before I lost the ability to move my legs, I had felt what I can only describe as a "pop" inside my body, like something had snapped. I fell to the floor gasping for breath and terrified because I couldn't move.

It all seems so dramatic now, but it was very real and devastating at the time. I pinpoint that moment as the moment my cancer was born.

It all made sense.

Every time I had a stressful moment from that moment on, my cancer symptoms would rear their head. When the stress eventually became too intense for my body to handle, the cancer grew exponentially.

I had reached a time when my initial treatments were nearly finished.

My radiation oncologist decided she wanted me to do the full 30 days of radiation instead of just the 25.

Unfortunately, on the evening of the 25th dose, I was no longer able to urinate.

By the time I realized what was going on, my bladder felt like a water balloon about to burst. The closest hospital was half an hour away.

It was the most uncomfortable and painful car ride of my life!

By the time we got to the ER, I was screaming in pain.

I entered the ER stumbling and yelling that my bladder was blocked.

They rushed me into the back where I sat on a port-a-potty, trying desperately to pee while the nurses scrambled around doing whatever it was they were doing. They got me on the gurney and tried to catheter me, but it wouldn't go in. After the third attempt, they got it through. Relief was slow, and I continually screamed that it wasn't working. One of the nurses said it should be subsiding, but it took ages before it did.

Apparently, my urethra had gotten clogged with crystalized, dead, white blood cells from the radiation. I also had cystitis, which was similar to a bladder infection, but not an infection. All of this was from the zappings. I had decided I wasn't going to do the last five doses of radiation.

When things calmed down and I was in the ER room by myself, the doctor finally came in.

He pulled up a seat and sat next to me.

Our conversation was something that would stick with me throughout the duration of my treatments and change forever how I viewed my situation, as well as how I viewed Western doctors in general.

Here's how the conversation went.

DOCTOR: You're the same age as me. How did you get this?

ME: It was stress.

DOCTOR: (shaking his head) I don't buy that. Lots of people have stress.

And he walked out of the room.

I don't think I was in shock over the abruptness of how the conversation ended so much as why it ended. He made up his mind that I wasn't credible and no more discussion on it was needed.

The truth is, I was so used to doctors treating me as if what I had to say about anything (including my own body) didn't matter, that I initially shrugged the incident off. It wasn't until I started researching it, and finding out that there were other people, AND other doctors who were starting to believe stress was a real cause of illness, that I started getting angry about his presumptuous ignorance. I was angry about ALL doctors who were ignorant. It was my body, and this doctor, like so many before him, presumed to know my body better than I did. Just because he knew how the endocrine system worked didn't mean he knew how MINE worked. Doctor's know the general function of human systems, but they don't know our individual bodies. Not even close.

Here I will take a small break away to mention that during my treatments, David exhibited symptoms similar to mine on several occasions. The doctors thought that he was having sympathy pains seeing what I was going through, and he probably was in some ways. We later found out that he had a little something of his own going on, but the point of this story is that one of the urgent care doctors we saw for David said the most intelligent thing I'd ever heard a doctor say that I wish all doctors lived by. He said, "The patient is their own best doctor. No one knows their body better than they do."

These words have become my number one motto and I believe they are a very strong reason why I've survived. They're words that gave me strength when I had to make my own choices that weren't exactly what the doctor's wanted.

The ER sent me home with the catheter still inside my bladder draining, telling me to go to an urologist in three days to have it changed.

The very next day, when I was supposed to be getting another radiation dose, I met with the radiation oncologist instead. I told her there would be no more Star Trek Enterprise rides for me (the radiation machine makes the same sounds as the starship on that show). She insisted I do the last five zappings, and promised that they would be more focused on the tumor, and that there would be no more bladder involvement, at all.

I asked her how important she really felt they were, and she said they were detrimental.

So I did them.

Meanwhile, I had to get the bladder catheter removed. The urologist put a fresh one in, and told me my bladder had to heal before I could ditch the catheter. It was horribly painful being cathetered again and I highly recommend avoiding the experience if at all possible. In hindsight I wouldn't have let them do it. My bladder got lazy after being cathetered for so many days and threatened to not work at all on its own after that.

Finally, my treatments ended. It should have been a time to rejoice, but immediately afterwards, the Witch Creek fires came through, and forced us to evacuate the farm.

Before we left, we tried desperately to get all the animals into a huge enclosed trailer to be relocated. Between my landlords, David, me and one or two other people, we got most of the animals inside it. Some went easier than others.

It's a testament to what the human body can do when a crisis presents itself.

As exhausted and worn out as I was from my

treatments, my landlord and I forced a 400 pound donkey up the ramp and into the trailer. She pulled on the reigns as I pushed from the back. That animal had all four legs out in front of her and was in no way, shape, or form, going into that trailer by her own free will.

By the time we were able to leave, we could see the flames on the ridge just above our property. The Sheriff had to escort us out, and we had to leave all of our chickens, the emu, the really big donkey, and a couple of llamas. Even the beautiful black swan had to be left behind.

In town, the ash and smoke was thick, and the traffic had us stalled for two hours. Ramona is a small town in the San Diego foothills with only three ways out and the fire had one completely blocked off. We knew it wouldn't be long before one of the others was blocked, too.

By the time we decided we couldn't leave town on the San Diego road, and the only other road we could, the flames were over the ridge, and not half a mile from the main road we were on.

The road was completely deserted going down the hill. David was in his car, and I was behind him in mine.

I was so scared the flames were going to catch up with us. It was even scarier when we reached the bottom of the pass and saw about ten fire trucks on the side of the road with their lights flashing just waiting for the town to be evacuated so they could go up.

David and I spent 7 days at my Mother's house thirty miles away while the fires consumed nearly everything in the county. More fires sprung up, and the one we had run from nearly reached us where we were.

When we were finally allowed to go back home on the

eighth day, we didn't know whether our farm and remaining animals had been consumed, or not.

In the end, the fire had reached the backyard of our landlord's house before splitting off and going around the property, then meeting up again, and raging down the Pasqual pass that we had used to get out.

It was heartbreaking that all our neighbor's homes and farms had been consumed by fire all around us, but we were thankful our house was just a sooty mess that needed to be cleaned up and not a single one of our animals died. Maybe it helped that our landlord was the former chief of the San Diego fire department.

Twelve weeks later, I went in for my colon resection/gallbladder removal, right at the beginning of the New Year of 2008.

The night before the surgery, a wound-ostomy nurse called me. She informed me that she would be the one who would teach me how to change my ileostomy bag after the surgery.

Wait...what? Ileostomy? What the hell is that???

She apologized that she had to be the one who told me. Someone else should have told me weeks ago. Well, yeah...that would have been nice information to prepare for! The last I heard, I wasn't going to need one of those. Okay, so I'm not getting a colostomy. What's the difference between an ileostomy and a colostomy?

Colostomy as described earlier: A portion of the intestine that sticks out of the body, diverting waste into a poop bag that's glued onto the side of the body. The difference between this and an ileostomy is that an ileostomy is the small intestine, not the large intestine, therefore stools are much more watery, and one cannot control when waste is going to come out. Not Webster's definition, but you get the point.

I was horrified.

It made it just slightly less horrifying that it wasn't going to be a permanent fixture.

Dr. R. informed me the day of surgery that I'd only have it for two or three months, at the most. Just until the intestines healed from the resection surgery, then she'd reconnect me.

Okay, I could deal with that, I thought.

The day of the surgery was something I barely recollect.

I remember waking up after the surgery feeling crazy. There was activity all around me with people rushing around asking each other for something, or other.

I could hear them talking about giving me another blood transfusion, and talking about whether or not the blood had been irradiated. Then I lost consciousness again. I remember next seeing David walking around the foot of my bed, and my Mom sitting in a chair in the corner, reading. Then I saw the outline of a huge pink elephant above her head. Wow! People really do see pink elephants! I just saw the outline of one, though. I saw a couple of other weird things that night that I don't remember now.

I remember feeling my body with my hands at some point.

My mid-section was tightly wrapped up in some sort of shapewear. I felt instantly relieved to know that I was swaddled so well. At least I felt confident that my guts weren't going to fly out at any moment. And that's exactly how it felt. My body knew it was in pieces being held together by stitchings of string, and maybe a few staples here and there, but not much more.

The next eight days were challenging to be sure.

The nurses tried to get me walking on day three, and it was very difficult.

Despite the pain in my tailbone that had been more painful than just about anything, it really did feel like my guts were going to spill out.

I began refusing to walk as much as they wanted me to. I knew it was good for the healing process, but it was just too painful. Sleeping was out of the question because the tailbone pain would get so bad I'd have to try and shift my weight from one hip to the other to alleviate some of it, and I just couldn't move very well. Also (and anyone who's ever spent a night in the hospital knows this), the nurses come in every hour to take vitals, and I was NEVER able to sleep through that.

I wasn't allowed to eat for the first six days, and I can't remember the reasoning behind that now. They might have been waiting for my bowels to wake up, but I was on a poop bag, so maybe I had to have a poop bag event. At any rate, when I was finally allowed to eat, I was so hungry, the cold, overcooked vegetables tasted like a gourmet meal!

I missed Rainbow and all the other animals so much. I just wanted to go home.

On the eighth day, I was paroled.

Home wasn't much comfort, though.

Trying to walk was an effort in futility and I wasn't able to change my ileostomy bag by myself. I had sutures from my pubis all the way up to the base of my chest, and I never wanted to remove the swaddle.

My Mother helped me every day, driving thirty miles

each way and without her, I might not have made it through those next two weeks.

David was the one who changed my poop bag except when I'd have an accident, like the bag leaking, or falling off when he wasn't around. Then I would do it myself, but I hated it. Sometimes the bag would burst in bed, and it was these moments that sent me into fits of tears. Still, David was a trouper and cleaned up my messes without complaint. I was feeling like such a big baby.

Eventually the abdominal wound healed, but the pain in my tailbone remained just as painful as ever. I knew something was wrong, but my oncology nurse would only suggest a chiropractor. This went on for months until I finally insisted on seeing a specialist. They referred me to another doctor who ordered a bone scan. She interpreted it as mild osteoporosis, or osteopenia, but said that shouldn't cause much pain. I was getting ready to do the adjuvant chemo, as my doctors all recommended, but I did it begrudgingly. It was going to be a hard road.

I was staged a IIIC, with four out of fourteen lymph nodes being positive, but margins around the tumor were negative for cancer, and the radiation had completely killed the cancer in the tumor.

The first chemo treatment immediately caused neuropathy in my hands, face, and legs. This caused a sensitivity to anything remotely cold. It felt like I was getting burned. I was terribly sick that whole week, then the second week was a little better. The treatments were in the cancer center in the infusion room, every two weeks. The first week was always the hardest, with the effects wearing off during the second week. The neuropathy got worse with each subsequent treatment and lingered longer.

If I drank anything that was room temperature, or colder, it would cause the sensation of my throat closing shut. The one thing I didn't have much of a problem with was nausea. Besides the neuropathy, the fatigue and fast exhaustion were the worst problems and I was getting through that okay.

Then another devastating blow happened.

A month after starting chemo, David and I got evicted from the farm.

I knew we weren't doing as good a job as if I were well, so I never blamed our landlords for doing it, but it was a very difficult thing. I suspected that David had said something to them. After all, he was doing most of the work there. I had been able to do some of it since recovering from surgery, but I wasn't able to lift much, and I was slow.

Our landlords mentioned in the eviction that David wasn't happy. That's why I suspect he said something to them.

I was so sad, but refused to let it ruin my life. Knowing the severity of my diagnosis helped me keep my mood upbeat. I just kept telling myself that every seemingly bad thing that has ever happened to me ended up having a positive outcome. This would be no different. I just couldn't see the positive outcome yet.

Meanwhile, the tailbone pain was increasing, and walking was nearly unbearable. Something was very wrong.

I finally insisted on getting a referral to a bone specialist.

The osteopath diagnosed me with nearly off the chart severe osteoporosis. He showed us on the scan the little

45

lines through the bones that he suspected might be bone metastasis, too. He ordered an MRI which took a week to schedule, and then another week after that before I could see the doctor.

Wow! WHAT a nerve-wracking two weeks THAT was!

I hadn't experienced many feelings of doom since diagnosed with cancer the year earlier, but when the suggestion of bone metastasis came up, I was sent into a panic.

I looked everything up I could online about bone metastasis. It didn't look good, not good at all, but I immediately began searching for people who survived a bone mets diagnosis. Yes, there were people who had.

I immediately went into plan mode. In other words, I made out a plan on how I was going to eat, what I was going to read, and everything else I was going to do in case it did come back as bone mets.

The MRI, thankfully, came back showing there were no bone mets. The lines on the bones were insufficiency fractures, or small breaks caused by a weakness in the bone. Well no wonder I could barely walk anymore!

I knew immediately the weakness in the bones was from the radiation treatments, though most of my doctors would blame the chemo, there were known instances of radiation causing insufficiencies in bone. It wasn't common, of course. I always seemed to fall within the slim part of the odds. Rare to get colorectal cancer under the age of 40, rare to get osteoporosis and insufficiency fractures from radiation...hopefully I would also fall within the slim part of the odds for survival, too.

As far as our moving from the farm was going, David and I had very few options.

46

We had no money for a move. SSI kept denying my application for one reason or another, and David's wages were not enough to support the two of us.

His Mother had been asking us to move in with her for some time, so that was the decision we made. David's oldest brother also lived there.

It was very hard leaving the farm, but I got along well with David's Mother, and it seemed like it could end up a better situation in the long run. Again, knowing my illness was triggered by stress, I tried very hard to see it all as a positive thing. I thought David's Mother and I could help take care of each other, and I wouldn't have the stress of taking care of a farm I simply wasn't capable of handling anymore. David's Mother was getting on in years, and David's brother wasn't exactly healthy, either. Another benefit was that we would be living twenty minutes closer to my cancer center, and David's job.

So a month after starting chemo, we moved.
May, 2008.

I should have gotten the ileostomy reversed around this time, but it was decided (by my doctors) that we would wait until I had finished my six months of chemo before undergoing another surgery.

I didn't like that idea, at all!

The ileostomy was the bane of my existence. I didn't understand how anyone could live their whole lives with one, but I knew people did it all the time. It was probably just another example of a seemingly negative situation becoming a positive one. Heck, no more urgent bathroom issues and abdominal cramps for them!

I got to the point where I was capable of changing the poop bag myself, but I let David do it most of the time, anyway. It just gave me the creeps unimaginably. Seeing a part of my INTESTINES sticking out of a hole on the side of my body...I just couldn't get passed it.

When chemo finished in August, I immediately set to work on getting the ileostomy reversed. I found out while checking in for an appointment that my insurance had dumped me.

I had been picked up by Medi-Cal (California Medicaid) shortly after my diagnosis, and after my adjuvant chemo ended, they decided I no longer needed them. Without needing a doctor to deem me in remission, or cured, they just decided on their own that I was healed.

This sent me into an hysterical panic.

I called everyone I could to try and get it reinstated, but since I hadn't been deemed disabled, and I wasn't under 21, or over 65, and wasn't blind, it wasn't happening.

I had been denied SSI several times, but kept appealing their refusals. According to their own rules, they couldn't take away benefits while it was in the appeals process. Someone decided to over-look that rule.

A lengthy struggle ensued, and I was unable to get the ileostomy reversed, or any medical treatments for my other issues, either. I had gained 70 plus pounds during chemo, and had developed diabetes as a result. I could barely walk with the fractured tailbone, and was taking an osteoporosis drug and a diabetes drug that I could no longer afford without the insurance. I was a waif in the wind; abandoned to die a slow and meaningless death! I'm over-dramatizing, but that was surely how I felt at the time. I knew the odds of becoming a stage IV were not good for someone in my position, and I would need to be watched very closely to catch anything life-threatening.

48

Was I going to have to live my life worrying about every little pain and change that popped up without being able to have it checked? If I got my health insurance back was I going to have to remain stressed out that medical treatment could be denied to me at any given second?

I had had enough.

I started reading health books and watching videos about people who cured themselves of cancer with and without traditional treatments. I had always been an occasional health fanatic. I was a vegetarian for more than a decade before my diagnosis, but it was for ethical reasons above anything else. I went back and forth between vegan, raw, lacto-ovo, and vegan again, all the time. I was interested in always eating healthy, but easily fell back into old habits of greasy, high fat foods. Still, I read everything I could on various diets. I had met a couple of people in one of my cancer support groups who claimed their cancers were cured with lifestyle change, alone. I was a woman without a purpose who was going to create one. Number one; find out how to take care of, and heal myself, by myself!

Thanks to Ellen, my psychology intern at the cancer center, I was able to get my Medi-cal reinstated, and it was almost business-as-usual. Until...

The insurance refused the ileostomy reversal, claiming it was an elective surgery! ARGH!!! Sigh...ARGH!!! Come on, really?

I was so tired of it all. Not only did I have to fight my own body, but the damn bureaucracy as well!

February, 2009.

After 14 months of struggling and fighting, and beating down the system, I was able to schedule the ileostomy reversal.

Then another problem reared its beautiful, cancer-loving head.

I was all prepped for the takedown surgery, wheeled into the operating room, and knocked out. I was so excited to finally be free of the poop bag, I was surprised the anesthesia worked at all! When I woke up, the first thing I did was feel around my body for the signs of the surgery. Instead of wearing that ole familiar, comforting swaddle wrap, I was wearing....AN ILEOSTOMY BAG!!

They were unable to do the reversal!

I kept asking angrily in a drug induced stupor, why I still had the bag, but no one would answer my slurred questions.

They wheeled me into the recovery room where Dr. R. informed me that
she couldn't do the reversal because there was a very tight, anastomotic stricture in my colon at the surgical site.

I had NO idea what that meant, or why they didn't fix it while I was under anesthesia, but I was too crushed to ask any more questions.

She explained that a stricture was a narrowing of the colon caused by scar tissue.

She said she had used a balloon dilation to expand the stricture, but could only get it to 14 mm, or something like that, and that it would have to be dilated to at least 20 mm before she could do the reversal.

^()&)(*^(&*)T^(^)(&%%*(&)^%$%! Those are cuss words, or any other available expletives to try and convey what I was feeling at that moment.

Oh, but wait, it gets better. There is salt in that wound..

Two hours after the failed surgery and all the

anesthesia had worn off, they took me to a procedure room where a GI doctor attempted to dilate the stricture some more.

The pain was some of the worst thus far. Possibly similar to a jailhouse rape where one performs the rape, and the others hold you down. I really wish I was exaggerating here.

I squeezed the nurse's hand until I thought I might have hurt her. I screamed and cryied that they shouldn't do that type of procedure without anesthesia. When he didn't stop, I punched him in the stomach. It wasn't out of malice. The shock of the pain caused me to instinctively turn and fight what was causing it. I did the same thing when I broke my arm at age ten and the doctor set the bones without any anesthesia. The difference between this time and that time, aside from the different ends of the body, was that the bone doctor warned me it was going to hurt. His exact words were, "this is going to hurt REALLY BAD".

After all of that, the GI still couldn't get the stricture open past 18 mm. I was going to need another dilation a month later, and I had to do it with this horrible doctor! I wasn't sure if it was worth it, and I didn't know why they weren't letting me use Dr. Moore, but I kept asking for him.

May 2009.

Finally, after two more dilations, the 15 month old ileostomy, the second worst torturer of my existence next to that GI doctor, was reversed!!!

I don't like being so dramatic about the ileostomy. There are many people who live happy, productive lives with permanent ones. I know I would have eventually

51

gotten used to it, but I can only imagine it would've been a very challenging road that would have taken a lot out of my quality of life. I was so overweight the bag never fit well and would fall off a lot. The other major downer was that my favorite thing to do was swim and I had major problems with the bag every time I went swimming or took a bath. It would not have been a high quality of life for me to have lived with an ileostomy. A colostomy would have been a much different story, as they are lower down on the large intestine, and can be better controlled. At any rate, I would advise anyone dealing with an ostomy to seek emotional support for it. Especially if you feel anything like how I felt about it. As my story goes, even after my nightmare experience with the ileostomy, I did consider getting a permanent colostomy not long after the reversal.

The time immediately following the takedown was like being back in the days before my diagnosis.

The stricture wouldn't allow ANYTHING to pass through the intestines easily. If I had too much liquid, the stricture wouldn't open up and allow that liquid to pass. It would stay trapped behind it causing miserable cramps. If I had too much fiber, the same thing would happen; nothing goes through. The abdominal cramping would cause such terrible pain in my tailbone I couldn't walk, sit or stand after just a few times of this.

Those early initial months after the reversal were very, VERY difficult. I was on a wound vac for the first four weeks, which is a pump attached to a tube that was attached to a sealed, water tight bandage on the wound that sucked out all the fluid and puss collected in the open wound. The wound couldn't be stitched shut for risk of infection, so there was a gaping hole in my abdomen that led straight to my intestines. It was probably about five inches deep, or more. Talk about living in a grossed out condition constantly! I could barely stand myself!

A nurse or two came to the house every day to change the bandaging, which was a welcome relief to me, and probably to David, as well!

The bathroom issues kept me pretty much in the house, except for doctor appointments.

When the wound healed enough, I began getting regular dilations for the stricture. The first two were with the doctor I couldn't stand until I was finally able to change to another doctor who was the complete opposite of the crappy one, AND she was female. I liked that.

As I mentioned before, the conscious sedation drug that is used as an amnesiac never worked on me. I always liked being able to remember what was done to me during those less invasive procedures. I always remembered everything, unless they gave me too much of it.

That happened once, and I spent the whole rest of the day vomiting.

The next time I came in for a dilation, I told her she had given me too much anesthesia, and to please not do that again.

She told me I had begged them to give me more drugs because the pain was so horrible! Oh my, I didn't remember that!

I then asked her not to listen to me if I begged for more drugs.

I was conscious through the procedure, and she was very gentle. The balloons are gauged only up to a certain amount of millimeters, so she had to change balloons after every couple of millimeters to dilate passed that. She did this very slowly until I couldn't stand the pain anymore, and then we pushed a little passed that.

After three of these procedures, I realized they really weren't helping me. I'd just be bowel incontinent for two or three days, then right back to being strictured again. I knew there had to be another way.

My best friend, Aaron, worked for one of the leading health food/raw food companies in the country and he was always bringing me great books and great supplements that had to be sampled. One day, he brought a large array of books for me that were mostly cancer centered, or about eating to cure and prevent cancer. I will list this company and their information in the appendix.

I sucked up the information like water to a sponge.

When I was done with those, I began researching everything I had read online.

Many of the books spoke about probiotics and how important they were in balancing the flora and fauna of our intestines.

I went out and bought myself a large bottle of Kefir, and drank it down.

The next day, I had an almost normal stool!!

This just motivated me to do more.

I started preparing raw food all the time and trying different types of probiotics.

My bathroom issues didn't go away, but the probiotics changed the dynamics of the problems tremendously. There were still other problems going on with the bathroom issues and the bone pain as well, but it was the beginning stages of learning how to take control of my own body and health. With each new discovery came a renewed energy and belief that I could heal myself completely.

3.
A TUMOR FOR ALL SEASONS

September, 2009.

David and I had gotten a portion of my medical records for some reason or other from the hospital. I was still in a battle with SSI, and there was now an attorney on it. This might have been why we got the records.

I had been reading through them when something caught my attention.

There had been a small mass found on my left lower lung that the radiologist and my colorectal surgeon both believed was metastasis.

The date the lesion was found was around November, 2008. Well here we were in the 9th month of 2009, and no one had ever mentioned anything about a lung mass to me!

I was both shocked and devastated.

This put me in an entirely different position as far as surviving the disease, and that was more than a slightly important thing to know.

When I brought this issue to my oncologist's attention, he was not at all concerned with it. He explained that the lesion hadn't changed much in the last several scans. Well, in one scan it appeared to be slightly larger, but different CT scans catch different angles of a mass, or whatever, and he just didn't think it was cancer. At any rate, we would keep an eye on it, and see.

I trusted him, but I was honestly disconcerted. I didn't feel comfortable questioning him too much about this. I had seen in the past where doctors would get huffy about their "expertise" being questioned by a patient. It had happened to me before, and I received quite a stern lecture about how much schooling the doctor had gone through to know better than I about something I had read on the Internet. I did, however, ask my oncologist to do a PET scan on it. He told me it was too small for a PET scan. I then asked for a biopsy, to which he explained that was too invasive of a procedure for something that was most likely nothing.

Colorectal cancer has many places it likes to spread in the body, but none are more favored than the liver and the lungs. I knew this. I'm pretty sure he did, too. Two other doctors, one an expert on reading CT films, and the other a highly respected surgeon, both believed it was metastasis. I couldn't understand why my oncologist wasn't being more pro-active about it. He was sure it wasn't cancer, and I wanted to believe it, too. So that's where we left it.

Little did I know I was in for another major life changing event that shifted my concerns into a completely new direction.

A month after our discovery of the lung lesion, David decided he wanted to end our relationship.

It was quite out of the blue and surprising.

I spent an hour wandering around his Mother's neighborhood trying to make sense of it and trying to come up with a plan of action just to cope with it.

I couldn't figure out what had happened. I blamed the cancer, and I blamed the diet changes I had made. I could tell David hadn't been happy with all the raw meals I was preparing, but I knew that couldn't be all of it. We were both vegetarians, so the raw change-over wouldn't have been that big of a deal. Whatever his reasons were, he wouldn't really elaborate. All I knew is that it was over, and another huge upheaval was going to happen in my life.

As painful as it was, I didn't fight him on it much. It wasn't at all like me. I was long ago disgusted by society's support of disposable relationships and always believed in doing everything possible to salvage a relationship before throwing it all away over frivolity.

For some reason, it really felt like the relationship had simply run its course and I had to do the next thing I had to do on my own, without him.

The last week of October, 2009, David helped me move into my grandmother's house, and that was the end of that.

4.
ANOTHER BEGINNING

It would have been the perfect situation as my grandmother was getting on in years and really needed someone to live with her.

The very night I moved in, she had a fall.

It wasn't the first time she had had one. In fact, she had had another fall a few days earlier that hurt her worse than the family realized. She should have been taken to the hospital that day, but she wasn't.

By the time Halloween came a few days later, my grandmother was able to get herself up okay, and seemed like she was fine.

On Halloween night, she fell trying to get herself to the port-a-potty next to the couch, and had to be taken to the hospital.

I had been out with some family members celebrating the Holiday, and my aunt was called to handle the incident.

At the hospital, they discovered that she had at least one cracked rib from the first fall, pneumonia, and was in active heart failure.

She spent the next month in a nursing home.

When she came home, she wasn't able to take care of herself anymore, at all.

I took care of my grandmother night and day for the next seven months. The pressure was grueling. Not just from being responsible for an entire other person, but from the pressure my aunt put on me to be responsible for everything my grandmother needed. They didn't want me leaving her alone, and getting people to relieve me once in a while wasn't easy. I was left with feelings of guilt if I had to go somewhere for even a few minutes. It was too much for me from day one, but there was no one else to do it.

There were days when it was very rewarding, and there were days when I thought I would have a nervous breakdown. My grandmother was feeble, incontinent, and stubborn about following rules such as not getting out of bed and wandering around the house in the middle of the night.

Many nights I couldn't sleep for fear I wouldn't wake up when she needed me. There was more than one instance when I got up in the morning, and found her lying on the floor because she had fallen in the night. There was no way I could get her off the ground once she was there unless I could get her into a position where she could hoist herself up. The osteopath had warned me that my spine was brittle on the inside, and could snap if I bent over to pick something up. This thought was always in the back of my mind whenever I bent over for something. Most times when she fell, I would get the fire department out there so they could put her back in bed.

She was on lots of meds that had to be given three or four times per day, and they had to be hand fed to her because we found out she had been missing doses when they would slip through her fingers trying to medicate herself. The chemotherapy had definitely done a number on my brain functioning and remembering to give her her meds was a struggle every day. Any doctor that says chemo-brain doesn't exist should give himself a chemo treatment or two, then give us his medical opinion!

Probably the most stressful aspect about the whole situation was the fear that my grandmother would die and it would be my fault somehow; whether I'd over-medicated her, or because she fell during the night. For the above reasons, coupled with the lingering threat of a cancer recurrence hanging over my head, I feared I had more than enough stress to cause the cancer to come back.

I constantly tried to keep myself in a happy, motivated state of mind. Sometimes I just HAD to get out of the house for some relief. I would sneak out to buy groceries late at night, or go for a walk after I had built myself up enough to do that. Each time, would be a workout of worry. What if she got up and broke her neck while I was gone? What if someone found out I had left her? My family would KILL me, and my own guilt would kill me!

Other family members were feeling stress from their own obligations to my grandmother, and began taking it out on me. There were verbal fights that sometimes culminated into screaming. Not just between my aunt and me, but between my aunt and my Mother and sometimes with my aunt and grandmother. Even though these events didn't happen often, I never knew when they would so I lived in fear of them.

The bathroom issues weren't helping anything, either. When the stress got even a couple of points above normal, I would be in the bathroom the better part of the day, and/or night, with painful cramps, diarrhea, or constipation. Bending over, or having to push or pull anything triggered bathroom issues and tailbone issues, too. I had a medical license to use marijuana, and some nights, it was the only way I could sleep without being awakened from the tailbone pain. I did this as rarely as possible for fear if something happened while I was under the influence, I'd go to jail.

My life had become nearly unbearable in seven, short months.

It was absolutely no surprise when they found the cancer had spread to an ovary in April of 2010.

I was going to need another surgery, and fast.

The issue of who was going to take care of my grandmother while I was in the hospital and then during my recovery, was a big question.

My Mother and aunt both had full time jobs. My cousin was married, and my brother worked six days per week. Besides all that...no one else wanted to do it.

They decided to hire an agency to send in workers for 24/7 shifts. It would be expensive, but there really wasn't any other choice short of putting my grandmother into a nursing home.

The docs also found that I had a major abdominal hernia, probably because of the stricture and bathroom issues. This would require a different type of surgery, and a different type of doctor.

In all, there would be three doctors present during the surgery.

Dr. R. would go in there and separate some adhesions that had formed and was a big contributor to my pain problems, and an OBGYN surgeon would remove both the ovaries. A general surgeon would repair the hernia.

Originally the plan was to give me a full hysterectomy since the odds were high I would someday develop some kind of gynecological cancer from all the radiation I'd had. That idea was nixed because the radiation had fused my uterus to my bladder, and the bladder would have had to been removed, too. They decided to take both ovaries instead.

The surgery was another success.

The general surgeon told me the hernia was more like seven hernias. So many, he could put his entire arm up into my abdominal and chest cavity. He put in a mesh that caused my body to be misshaped, but that was okay. It was never "in" shape to begin with. The adhesion surgery eventually took some cramping away. The OBGYN doctor did not take the good ovary as planned, and for a long time I was upset about this. Especially because the healthy ovary didn't look all that healthy to my oncologist and he wanted it removed. That would've meant yet another surgery.

The OBGYN doctor refused to remove it.

I can now thank her for that. The ovary was still producing needed hormones, and she disagreed with my oncologist. She thought it wasn't in that much danger of becoming cancerous.

Sometimes, all doctors have to do is trust their patients and tell them the reasoning behind their advice or decisions. In turn, it's up to us as patients, to voice our disagreements if we have any, and ask for the doctors reasoning.

It took me a very long time to learn how to stand up for myself when I thought a doctor was wrong. And believe me, they are wrong a lot. They are, after all, human.

5.
A BRAND NEW BODY; A BRAND NEW LIFE!

The ovary removal, or salpingo oopherectomy, as they like to call it, had me in the hospital for only five days. Generally they keep you in there until you pass gas, or poop. I passed gas fast because I wasn't interested in being starved again.

I felt so good, even with another huge abdominal wound. Most of the nerves at the surgical site had been completely severed from the first surgery, so I didn't feel much in the way of wound pain. That was both a blessing and a curse.

I burst several stitches, and the wound didn't heal right. That was okay. At least there was no infection, and no pain.

I was feeling so good, in fact, I had no desire to go back to taking care of my grandmother! At least not right away. I was ready to have a life! I felt like I hadn't really had a life in years, and I really hadn't!

I had lost a lot of weight, about thirty pounds at that point, and summer was coming. The weather was really warm by the time I had healed enough to be active, and I wanted to have some fun.

My life-long weight problem had kept me away from areas where less clothing was mandatory, so places like water parks and beaches had been off limits to me for years. Well, not anymore!

The first water park I went to was a small local one. That trip started an avalanche of water park trips all over two counties that summer.

It was great and I was physically enjoying life. Something I thought I'd never do again.

I went back to caring for my grandmother three days per week. Every, single, thing had to be done for her (even butt wiping), but thank goodness I had someone who came to shower her three days per week. Besides the hard work caring for her entailed, it was hard watching her deteriorate so slowly.

I still carried the heavy burden of fearing I would do something wrong and inadvertently cause her demise.

Every time something new was added to her regime (which happened often), it made it scarier and scarier.

At the same time, I was struggling to take care of myself both mentally and physically. I was putting a lot of effort into teaching myself how to deal with my stress and how to let go of past issues and bad habits so I could heal.

I had refused the doctor's recommendation to do chemotherapy treatments for my new stage of cancer, and was going it pretty much alone.

My oncologist was very displeased with my decision, but I had put in the needed time to do the research, which had started back in 08, and I truly believed that more chemo would do more harm than good.

It was a decision I had actually made before even starting the adjuvant chemo treatments back in 2008: my plan was to take all their poisonous chemo and radiation at first, but if the cancer ever came back, I would not go that route again. And I didn't.

The thing that really cinched that idea for me came after I had already done the six months of chemo treatments, and my oncologist informed me that there wasn't any evidence either way whether chemo worked, or not! What a fine how-to-do was that?

It strengthened all the reports and videos I had seen about chemo and it's uselessness against cancer.

Now don't get me wrong. I am not totally against someone doing chemo or going with the standards of care. I'll go back to all of that in a later chapter. For now, I'm just rehashing what I went through within myself.

I strongly believed that doing chemo would take away from my quality of life while I slowly died of the disease.

I had seen so many people in my online support group wither away after years of struggling with recurrence after recurrence, surgery after surgery, and chemo regime after chemo regime, only to end up dead. And it wasn't necessarily the cancer that was killing them. It was organ damage, or pneumonia, or some other lasting factor that the long-term TREATMENTS had caused.

I had clear memories in my head of when I first started chemo and the HAZMAT kit they equipped me with to use in case the chemo ever spilled out of my pump. I remembered when I had spilled some chemo on my nightgown, and the people I called to report it to told me to wash my nightgown several times, and use the gloves and disposable HAZMAT materials in my kit to clean it off the floor. This was stuff they were pumping constantly into my body, but outside of my body it was treated like the Chernobyl nuclear disaster!

It didn't make any sense to me that something that

toxic and poisonous could kill the cancer and not kill me in the process.

So I kept refusing the chemo every time I saw my oncologist for follow-ups. I was getting scanned every three months and so far coming up pretty clean.

Did I mention that I felt really good?

Aside from the bathroom issues that were still a constant problem, and the fractured tailbone that made certain activities impossible, I learned to be somewhat happy, and somewhat active in my life.

My grandmother's condition would improve, then worsen, then improve again.

The caregiver who came four days per week really lessened the stress on me, but still kept me confined to the house three days per week. My grandmother had been in hospice care ever since returning from the nursing home in 2009. On my days when she was bowel incontinent were probably the worst for me as far as trying to clean her up and there was no way I could do a good enough job, but luckily those days were not common.

This continued throughout the rest of 2010.

I had started dating again around August of that same year for the sheer purpose of wanting to get out and feel normal again. It was great entertainment, too. I NEVER expected to find Mr. Right. Heck, I had stopped believing there was such a thing as a Mr. Right long before I even met David!

Dating again definitely helped me feel somewhat normal, but it also gave me the grim realization that I probably would never experience romantic love again. I was fairly certain no one would want to get that deeply involved with someone with as serious an illness as I had, and I definitely didn't want the heartache when he found out he couldn't handle it.

I had met a man who was a colorectal cancer survivor, too, who was the same age as me. He had already been NED (no evidence of disease) for ten years. He had been diagnosed a stage III.

I dated him for about a month, and thought he was just the sweetest guy. And he was...there was just absolutely NO SPARK. In fact, I couldn't stand to date him any longer because I felt he really liked me and I knew in my heart the relationship could never go any further than friends.

Most of the other men I dated I liked much less. Except for one other whom I got along with really well and had tons of stuff in common with, but I still only wanted to be friends with him.

In March of 2011, everything, and I mean EVERYTHING, changed.

I unexpectedly met a man I genuinely liked. In fact, I could picture myself falling head over heels for him. Uh-oh...better run now!

I didn't run, though I wanted to many times. He was smart, he was good looking, he was spiritual in the same ways I was spiritual, he was so many things that appealed to me, and...he really liked me to!

I had decided early on in dating that I would inform potential datees of my cancer situation. Many had run away with their tails between their legs right away. One of them even said to me, "well, what can you expect, it's scary." I had to agree with him, and on many occasions I thought it might be unfair of me to allow someone to care for me so much just so they could watch me die. But I

68

didn't believe I was going to die. At least I really felt I wasn't going to die of colorectal cancer. To me, my future was just as unknown as anyone's and I deserved to live that way.

A life coach by profession, Chris had seen a LOT in his life, more than enough, in fact, to prepare him for me.

He didn't run when I told him about the cancer.

He still didn't run when I told him about the stage and survival odds.

Instead, he lifted my spirits up, and made me want to live more than ever.

In those first few months of our relationship, he helped me through so much.

My aunt had pulled a fast one on me and was trying to manipulate me into doing what she wanted me to do in regards to my grandmother. It felt like there was constant conflict and butting of heads.

She wanted even more care for my grandmother by me, and it got to the point where she started to demand I work at least four days per week or I needed to find another place to live.

Things were getting so bad in the family, the greed and ulterior motives of certain family members could no longer be suppressed. It started with a "family meeting" where even the hired caregiver got involved in the disagreement and threw accusations of all kinds, for what purpose, I wasn't sure. My cousin and her husband got involved, too, again, for what purpose I didn't know. It became a fiasco of accusations that was pretty obviously stemming from the fact that I was refusing to work that fourth day. It didn't make much sense, but it didn't matter. All I knew is that I was sick to death of the bullying and having to explain myself to those who thought they had the right to demand anything at all from me. My living there and voluntarily caring for my grandmother was saving the family thousands of dollars per month, but yet it wasn't good enough for them. Thinking back on it, I suppose they thought I didn't have any recourse, or anywhere else to go. They were wrong.

Neither my grandmother, nor I, had been happy with the relief caregiver. We each had our different reasons, but after what happened with the "family meeting", my grandmother asked my aunt to get a different caregiver which of course should have been someone me and my grandmother chose since we were the two people who had to live with the choice. Of course my aunt refused to get rid of the woman, and she and her daughter spent 45 minutes bullying and brow beating my grandmother into not only agreeing with them, but into putting my greedy aunt in charge of all of her financial affairs. They didn't realize I could hear almost everything they said through my bedroom wall. Lies, guilt trips, and my pregnant cousin even going so far as telling my grandmother the situation was stressing her out (a situation that had absolutely nothing to do with her). The onslaught of harassment they gave her that day for their own selfish wants, not only surprised me (even after what they had already done to me), but it changed my entire perspective of how far self-righteous people will go to get what they want. I just couldn't believe my ears.

As soon as they left, I went out to collect my grandmother to put her to bed, and to apologize to her for what they had done. I had no sooner got her to her feet when she became unresponsive and fell against me and pushed me into the entertainment center, pinning me . I couldn't get her to speak for a few minutes, and she was weak on one side of her face. I knew right away she was having a stroke, but when she came out of it I realized it had to have been a mini-stroke.

Almost immediately she told me she didn't want anything more to do in decision making with her affairs and that she just wanted peace in the family. My poor, old grandmother.

I reported the incident to hospice as elder abuse and asked them to document it, but since there was a conflict between the two sides of the family, I don't know if they believed me.

Not long after that, my aunt snuck an attorney into the house sometime while I was out, and had my grandmother change her trust to make my aunt the sole trustee of her will. I warned my mother that my aunt would most likely try something like that, but she didn't want to believe it. I understand the shock that ensues when you find out someone you would trust with your life is as dishonest and untrustworthy as a common criminal. It was exactly how I felt when I saw what my aunt had done and had continued to do.

I began concerning myself with escaping.

I found a room to rent in a nice house on the outskirts of town and was all ready to sign the rental agreement when some other family members talked me into staying at my grandmother's mainly for financial reasons. My grandmother was running out of money, and a full time caregiver couldn't really be afforded. It was the last thing on Earth I wanted to do, but it was more horrific for me to think that my grandmother would end up in a nursing home for her last days.

So I sucked it up, even though living there had become 200 times more difficult having to live there with the caregiver that had gotten involved in the family affairs, and still having to deal with those wicked family members who both repulsed me and made me uncomfortable. Trapped like a rat in a flooded sewer full of crap, my only solace was Chris. He kept my stress levels from giving me a heart attack with his encouragement and support.

Unfortunately, it wasn't enough to keep me healthy.

The stress had awakened a sleeping giant inside me. It had gathered its legions and was years beyond mad.

6.
ONE MORE GO, AND THEN GOOD-BYE

In October of 2011, it was discovered that the stable lesion in my lung (the one found back in 2008), had begun to grow suddenly.

By the time a CT scan was done to confirm its growth a month later, it had nearly doubled in size and had grown spindly (spikes all over it).

It was surely cancer, and it had to be taken care of immediately.

I was scheduled to see a pulmonologist the following week.

He decided a biopsy wasn't necessary. He just wanted to go in and get it ASAP. I strongly agreed with him.

He thought he could save the lobe, and just take out a wedge. This was also a huge relief.

If only life could be that easy.

In December, while checking in for pre-op evaluations, and only a week away from my scheduled surgery, we were informed that my insurance had changed and was no longer good at UCSD.

My normally low blood pressure began to rise. If I hadn't been experienced in these things by now, and if I hadn't been practicing controlling my stress levels, I might have gone through the roof. As it was, I pretty calmly began formulating a plan.

I called everyone I could think of at that very moment to try and fix it. I had programmed important phone numbers into my phone, and knew who to call.

I was really confused. I had government insurance, how could it change to private insurance?

Well, that's pretty much what had happened.

Apparently Medi-Cal had given me the choice to choose what medical insurance I wanted, and since I hadn't taken the time to figure it out, it chose one for me. What it chose was to remove me from insurance that covered UCSD, to some other that didn't. Probably a mindless decision of some bureaucrat, or maybe even a computer had done it. At that time, I didn't understand it. I didn't remember Medi-Cal giving me any choices to choose a health plan.

I felt for a moment like I was totally screwed.

I was desperate to get the cancer out of me. I already felt like this dip in the road was quite possibly my last. I understood what mitosis was (the rate at which a cell reproduces), and I was well aware of what an aggressive cancer could quickly do. Even though I didn't know the mitosis for this cancer, I knew it was faster than it had ever been before, and that's all I needed to know to know it had gone aggressive. I also didn't know for sure at this time whether it was more colorectal cancer spread, or a new primary of lung cancer.

It turned out that getting the insurance switched back to UCSD would've taken months and I wasn't guaranteed back in because there was a waiting list, or WHATEVER.

I was back to square one.

I made an immediate appointment with a new primary doctor for the very next day, and with her, made appointments with a new oncologist. That step alone put us into January, then meeting with the new pulmonologist, and new scans of the little bugger put us into February.

My surgery was finally scheduled for March 9th, and the time for a wedge-ectomy had long, since passed. The whole lower lobe would have to go. I kept my cool about it pretty well.

I can sit from this vantage point now and say it all worked out for the best, but I was really scared at the time. I didn't know what losing an entire lung lobe was going to do to my breathing capacity, and even though the doctor told me it wouldn't make much of a difference, just the fact that he added, "You're not a marathon runner, so there probably won't be much of a change," told me I'd probably notice a difference and it wouldn't be a small one.

As soon as I awoke from the surgery, I had my answer.

I could barely breathe and could only gasp for air. It felt like an elephant was sitting on my chest, when in reality, it was probably only a small cow. That was a joke. An elephant would've crushed me, but that's what was going through my mind at the time. Remember the pink elephant I saw during my first surgery? I think elephants are my spirit animal.

They put me in ICU with the nursing station right in front of me. I kept crying for them to help me, and they kept telling me there was nothing they could do. Every time I fell asleep I stopped breathing and a loud buzzer would startle me awake.

Those first two days were not fun.

When they moved me into my own room, things got better with the breathing. They were giving me breathing treatments regularly, and I was on oxygen.

The only major bummer was the drainage tubes in my side. They prevented me from being able to go anywhere and the nurses made sure I didn't try by putting an alarm on my bed. Every time I tried to go use the bathroom, a loud buzzer rang out. Now I knew how my grandmother felt!

Those tubes in my side were rubbing on something inside my body that caused a debilitating pain. I can only describe it as muscle seizures. It felt like the muscles in my abdomen were twisting and contorting. At first we didn't know what was causing it. When the doctors came and pulled the tubes out a few days later, the pain instantly ended, so I know the tubes had something to do with it. It happened again several times after that, so I don't know if the tubes injured something, or if it was just the change in my physiology. I was back in the ER a few days after being released from the hospital via ambulance because the contortions had me, well, contorted.

After the surgery, I got to go home on the fourth day. The shortest hospital-stay, ever! I was both relieved, and distraught.

I missed my animals, and was finally able to sleep, but I didn't know what hell awaited me at my grandmother's.

My aunt was pressuring me to move out. Apparently she had solved the financial dilemma of caring for my grandmother, and started putting the pressure on me to move a week after I got home.

She wanted to move a permanent caregiver for my grandmother into my room, even though there was another spare room in the house. What could I do? I had at least one broken rib, but most likely two from the surgeons spreading them apart to get to the lung, and I was, of course, in a lot of pain from it. I didn't think I would be able to move all my stuff, but nevertheless, I began moving into my Mother's house two weeks after surgery.

I can't express enough what an amazing relief it was once it was done, and I was moved out of my grandmother's house and out from under the control of my hateful aunt! It was a freedom I hadn't known in a long time. Even though I wasn't completely out, most of my stored stuff was in my grandmother's garage, and my cats had to be left temporarily, all I really cared about at the time was enjoying my new found liberty.

Unfortunately, my Mother's house was small and full of her own stuff. There wasn't any room for all the stuff I had in my grandmother's garage. While we were in the process of trying to make room, my aunt hired someone to take all of my stuff out of my grandmother's garage and stack it all in the side and front yards where many items "vanished" mysteriously, or were ruined right away because they were items that couldn't be left outside; like the washer and dryer. All of this so the caregivers could park their cars in the garage. Now I can tell you that in the 44 years I'd been alive, I don't recall anyone EVER using that garage to put a car in it! I guess my aunt figured just one more, wicked flexing of her muscles was warranted for me refusing her control. "How dare you go against my wishes you little ingrate!"

We hurried as fast as we could to rescue as much of my belongings as possible, but nearly all of it just ended up in my Mother's yard, where after many a rainstorm, found their demise as well.

It took me a year to be able to go out there and look at all the damage that had been done and to throw away the things that got ruined. I felt even more betrayed by my own family members seeing some sentimental items ruined, but once I let that go, and once I had the control to eliminate the abusive people from my life, that's when the real freedom took hold of me.

After that, I didn't have much of a problem throwing away the things that got ruined. I looked at it as a purge to begin a new life free of so many bits of junk I was holding onto for no real purpose.

I found some very positive things out of the experience. Moving out of my grandmother's house put me in the position I needed to be in, in order to heal from my cancer. That was the most positive thing ever. My grandmother was the real victim, no longer having someone who loved her living with her and aiding in her care was sad for her, I know it was.

Towards the end, I have the comfort of knowing that as her ability to identify people she knew faded, she always remembered who I was when she saw me, and her eyes always filled with joy.

I still have a lot of problems with the lobectomy surgery site, and I suspect that's because I wasn't able to heal properly from it, but that's a very small price I had to pay.

The lung margins came back clear, and the four lymph nodes they took
 surrounding the area also came back negative for cancer.

My new oncologist strongly recommended another six to eight months of chemo to make sure all the little straggler cancer cells were killed, but I graciously, and continually, decline.

I'm scanned every three or four months like clockwork, and probably will be for a good many years to come. My oncologist has stopped recommending chemo and agrees that if anything should pop up again, we'll treat it with surgery.

I remained NED for a couple of years after the lobectomy until Chris and I had a strange parting of ways that mirrored the situation that caused my cancer in the first place.

A few months after that, the PET scans began lighting up in the same exact area of my original tumor; just behind the anastomotic stricture.

Three GI doctors couldn't reach it to biopsy it, but when I went back to Dr. R., we found out that it was growing and was surely another recurrence.

Since so much damage had already been done to my intestines, I was not a candidate for another resection. Dr. R. wanted to start discussing another surgery to remove it and put me on a permanent poop bag. It wasn't a conversation I was willing to have. For me, this was just going to be another challenge I'd find my own way to deal with, and I did.

In the next few chapters, I'm going to share with you everything I've learned over the past ten years about how I believe I've kept my cancer from going crazy all over me without the use of harsh chemo treatments. Even though I've had three (unofficially, four) recurrences, the cancer was mostly a slow mover (until the lung met) that I was able to keep in check because of several factors. I think of it as a formula for my healing and it's a formula anyone can put into practice on their own terms. My hope is that a person dealing with cancer, or with any other illness, can design their own formula for healing and gain control of their disease, or even knock it completely out of the game on their own. Harsh chemicals are not the only choice AVAILBALE to us. They're the only choice GIVEN to us for a number of different reasons, but one major one I'll also discuss. Being a lay person with very limited medical training and only a certification in nutrition, I hope I can inspire others like me, to trust themselves and their bodies. A medical degree is not required to know and understand our own bodies.

I believe most, if not all, illness and disease is our body's way of telling us something in our lives isn't right. If we can locate and repair that first, the rest is easy. Discovering what that is can be challenging, rewarding, and exciting, but even if we never know 'why' cancer's entered our lives, I full-heartedly believe we can still turn it all around.

7.
TRIGGER HAPPY

In October of 2007, during my first chemo excursion, I joined an online support group for colorectal cancer survivors through the American Cancer Society's website called The Cancer Survivor's Network (CSN). The group of people on that site helped me more in understanding what was going on with my disease, and knew more of what I needed to expect than any six oncologists. The people there had answers for me when my doctors didn't, and sometimes even corrected wrong information the doctors gave me.

I suspected that stress was what caused my cancer. There was little doubt about it, but before my tumor was aged, it was still just a young thought in my head. When I posted this on the website, commenting about how I thought stress was a major factor, someone responded that she didn't care how she got her cancer, just as long as she got rid of it.

Her statement really got me wondering how important it was for me to know EXACTLY how, and why, I got my cancer. It was a short debate within me. Yes, it was very important for me to know how I got my cancer. How could I possibly cure it if I didn't change what caused it in the first place? I didn't know if it was possible. I didn't believe cancer just sprung up in me for no reason. Something somewhere, must have occurred differently to me that didn't occur to someone else. Though every person and every case is different, for me, there was a specific trigger, or one big, powerful thing that kick started my illness.

It took me a long time before I realized that cancer isn't just a disease. It's not just a civil war raging within our bodies; our own cells turning against one another where good cells can't tell themselves apart from the bad cells. I came to learn that cancer can have many different faces. It can be genetic in the form of FAP, K-RAS, or Lynch Syndrome to name a few. Some say it's a fungus, others a virus. I think it's possible that cancer can be all of those things, depending on the person, and what factors they have. To me, what it is wasn't nearly as important as to WHY it was there. I figured when I knew why it was there, I could change the environment of why it was there, and logically it would go away.

I learned all I could about cancer's likes and dislikes, and I could see that there were hundreds, maybe thousands of factors that contribute to cancer in simple, everyday life: Some big, some small, but all around us just the same.

I made a list of all the cancer factors I had in my own life that I was aware of, and was shocked to see how many there were. How many were probably in everyone's lives. I began to wonder why we ALL didn't have cancer! Then I learned that we all DO have cancer. Our bodies are usually able to destroy the mutant cancer cells faster than the cancer cells can gain control, in most cases, that is. In the cases where a person has detectable cancer, for some reason (and that reason for me was the trigger), the cancer was able to outsmart an overpower my immune system to grow basically unchecked as it pleased.

I'm not going to list every single factor that contributes to cancer, but I want to talk about a few that some of us don't even realize are a factor, but are probably contributing to our disease or weakened immune systems, nonetheless. Some of these may be controversial to some, but from my years of research, I believe they're all possible factors.

The factors I eliminated from my lifestyle are making a difference in keeping the cancer from completely overtaking me. Even if a person's trigger can't be easily identified, being conscientiously aware of the simple daily choices we make can make a big difference in our health and wellbeing. I know it has for me.

One factor is aluminum.

I believe aluminum is very dangerous and can cause all kinds of health issues, particularly colorectal cancer and Alzheimer's disease. It could be connected to breast cancer because of the aluminum in antiperspirants. It's also been linked to colorectal cancer in beluga whales who reside in the waters near an aluminum smelting factory (http://www.environmentalhealthnews.org/ehs/news/wildl ife-cancer).

I stopped buying deodorants that have aluminum in them and replaced all my pots and pans with stainless steel. I also avoid aluminum cans as much as possible, and always take any left overs out of the can before storing them in the refrigerator.

Microwave ovens.

In this day and age it's hard to imagine one's life without a microwave oven, but it is very possible and much safer to avoid them. Those of us born before 1980 can probably remember a time when we had to live without them.

I haven't completely eliminated the microwave oven from my life, but when it's running, I'm out of the room, far away from it. I also NEVER put food items in plastic in the microwave. This process can molecularly change the food. I don't see how that is a good thing. The only completely safe microwave is the one that isn't anywhere near you.

Chemically treated foods/GMO's.

I eat as organic as possible; especially soft skinned fruits and vegetables. There is a list of foods that should always be eaten unsprayed. I will include a list of these foods in the appendix.

I have read so many mixed opinions on whether or not organic is safer, or whether or not the certification is authentic, blar dee blar. I do the best I can with what's available near me. Of course growing my own food is a long term goal of mine, and will ultimately be the best choice, but realistically, not everyone can do that. As far as GMO foods, the word is out that they may not be safe and I say better safe than sorry. I avoid GMO foods as much as possible. If corn or soy is part of your diet, it will be hard to find these products that aren't GMO. I recently saw something that claimed Amish people have dramatically less cases of autism, ADHD, cancer, and other serious health issues that are plaguing us in this day and age, and it's suggested that this is because they don't use pesticides/herbicides, and do not have any GMO foods. I have seen two or three different articles on this, but I haven't read any actual studies. Just food for thought here (http://healthwyze.org/index.php/component/content/articl e/295-the-amish-dont-get-autism-but-they-do-get-bio-terrorism.html). I have read other possibilities why the Amish have lower rates of disease, and all probably play a part. All I know is it makes sense to eat as close to chemical-free as possible.

I use my better judgment when shopping for organic food, and when possible, shop as locally as possible. I avoid anything grown in Mexico or out of the country at all. The U.S. sells DDT and other poisons to third world countries such as Mexico and Chile to use on the produce they grow over there, then ship them over here for us to eat (http://npic.orst.edu/factsheets/ddtgen.pdf). Sheesh!

I've been reading tidbits of how food grown or produced in China is causing illness here in the U.S., since we get a lot of our food from over there. Even food that's supposed to be fresh, like fish, is coming from China! It takes two to four weeks to get a letter from China, there's no way I'm buying my food from there.

Fried foods. Yeah, I'm gonna take the fun out of everything!

A good motto to live by is; "if it's brown, turn it down". The browner the food, the less edible it is. This can even extend to breads and liquids, such as coffee.

Fried foods are carcinogenic. Barbecued foods, or anything charred is carcinogenic. Certain oils are more carcinogenic than other oils. Many oils used for cooking degrade quickly at high temperatures and become carcinogenic. Good oils to cook with are coconut, avocado, organic canola, and palm oil. Be conservative with these oils because some are highly saturated. A good alternative to oil in sautéing is balsamic vinegar and water with reduced sodium soy sauce. Baking is a great alternative to frying. Sprinkle a little coconut oil or coconut spray on whatever needs to be lightly crispy, and stick it in the oven. A touch of clarified butter is a good alternative to harmful oils, and much safer than margarine.

Margarine is one of the most unnatural substances on the planet. I don't
know what it is, and probably very few people could tell you. I believe margarine is the same as eating plastic: Avoid! Avoid! Avoid!

Other "food" ingredients that I eliminated, or avoid as much as possible are aspartame (chemical sugar alternative), anything hydrogenized, saccharine, and high fructose corn syrup. I got in the habit of reading labels on everything when I went vegetarian. After some practice, it got to where I knew instinctively what I did and didn't want, and reading labels is not as necessary. I have a rule I use with certain items that if there are more than four ingredients, or if there's anything difficult to pronounce in the listed ingredients, I don't buy it. Needless to say, I've gotten used to making my own meals from scratch. Like anything else, it just takes practice.

So much processed food barely resembles food at all. There's no nutritional value in it, and many of the ingredients were created in a lab.

More on oils.

I've heard so many conflicting things about oils, and it seems to be a controversial topic. Some nutritionists say canola oil, safflower oil, and "vegetable" oils are the worst as far as unhealthy oils go and should be avoided at all costs. I've heard others say these oils are great, and it's the high saturated oils such as coconut and palm that should be avoided.

From my own experience, and knowing the oils that degrade quickly with heat, I stay away from all oils except flax (which I use in salads, and on toast), cold pressed olive oil (mostly for salads), and sesame oil for Asian dishes quickly seared in a wok. For cooking, I only use coconut oil, which I believe is very healthy in small amounts, avocado oil, and organic, non-GMO canola oil. The research and opinions of others can be daunting, which is one reason why I've added a lot of my own personal experimentation on this matter, and the simpler I eat, the healthier it seems to be. If you don't know what it is (just what is "Canola", anyway), simply don't eat it (Canola is a flower). What is vegetable oil? That can be anything. I avoid it.

Another very controversial cancer factor is animal products in the diet. For me this is a no brainer. For others, messing with their steak is cause for a lynching! I would never tread on anyone's right to eat a dead animal, but hey, we're talking about eliminating factors that contribute to cancer here, and I'm not so sorry to say, there is enough evidence to prove animal products in the diet are unhealthy, though some are worse than others.

Most meat is loaded with toxins (antibiotics, hormones, they're fed animals of their own kind that died of diseases, etc.). Meat is also carcinogenic because of the way it's typically cooked. Grilled, barbecued, fried. If consuming meat is a necessity, a good idea would be to eat organic, grain-fed animals, and to bake, or broil it. Consume it in limited quantities, and no more than a couple of times per week. Also be very careful with fish, and remember that with fish, the lower on the food chain you eat, the less toxic the fish will be. Avoid shark, swordfish, and eat shellfish sparingly because of the heavy metals in them.

Heavy metals in our bodies can cause a plethora of damages, from brain function, to kidney function. I believe they can play a serious role in our ability to heal from disease, too, if they don't contribute to causing the disease in the first place. Heavy metals such as mercury, lead, arsenic, and aluminum are among the more common ones. Aluminum was the first factor I listed above, and as I've written, I believe it is the heavy metal most dangerous to those with colorectal cancer. The thing with aluminum is that it can be directly linked with CAUSING colorectal cancer if you read the study I sited above on the poor Beluga whales.

Chemotherapy has heavy metals in it, and is a big reason why the treatments damage organs. Heavy metals stay in the body indefinitely, sometimes forever, where they continually damage the body long after the cancer is gone. Heavy metals have been linked to Alzheimer's, Parkinson's, and MS (http://www.mindbodygreen.com/).

Amalgam, the metal used in dental fillings, contains mercury, which releases off-gases that constantly poison the body. Ocean fishes from all over the world, and particularly large fish and shellfish, all have varying levels of mercury and other toxic poisons in them. Store bought apple juice has been found to contain arsenic. Another great reason to stay away from processed foods. The good news about all of this is that there are natural ways to flush heavy metals from the body. The most natural way

I've heard of, is eating a lot of cilantro and/or coriander, and including a tablespoon of chlorella, or any kind of algae powder, mixed in water, juice, or whatever you like, per day to help reduce heavy metals in the body.

Dairy products also rank high on the cancer factor list. Like meat, they tend to have lots of toxins, antibiotics, and hormones in them. They produce a lot of mucous and inflammation in the body that can cause all kinds of health problems. If milk is a must, it's a good idea to use organic milk, but preferably rice, hemp, cashew or almond milk which are very good and healthy replacements and can be found inexpensively organic. I use cheeses in very limited quantities. The soft, white cheeses are probably safer than the orange, hard cheeses, and the yellow cheeses have rennet, which is acquired by pumping the stomachs of baby cows. Cheese is a serious weakness of mine, even more than chocolate, but I avoid it as much as possible. As of writing the second edition of this book, I have recently discovered that vegan cheeses are far superior to the ones from the 1990's, and are a wonderful replacement to dairy cheeses. They come in different flavors, and they MELT.

A word on chocolate; I believe dark chocolate is healthy. The darker the chocolate with the least amount of sugar in it, the better. In fact, the only thing harmful in chocolate is the sugar and milk (for humans, anyway. Dog's would disagree).

Some have come to believe, and I am among them, that gluten is a huge factor for causing colorectal cancer, if not in everybody, then for a lot of us.

I've been doing gluten experiments on myself for years and I'm convinced gluten is unhealthy and an unnecessary part of my diet. The stricture in my intestines made the experiments very easy. I eat gluten, I get an inflamed colon, and bathroom issues intensify. When I don't eat gluten at all, I feel less bloated, and have an overall sense of being lighter. Bathroom issues are just not as intense. I recently got complacent and ate flour tortillas for at least one meal for four days, and bread products during some of the other meals. Within a day I was back to having the same bathroom issues I had when the ileostomy was first reversed. I don't buy flour tortillas anymore.

I will get into more detail on gluten in the "To Eat, or Not to Eat" chapter. As for now, I will list it as a possible factor, and leave it up to the reader whether or not to eliminate it.

Vitamin D3 deficiency.

I have a very strong belief that this is a common factor many of us with cancer have. Whether it's a factor or a result, I don't know for sure, but some researchers believe there's a link between cancer and a D3 deficiency. There are a lot of articles and studies on the vitamin D deficiency and its link to various cancers, but I'm only going to site one of them (http://www.medicalnewstoday.com/articles/313933.php)

I didn't realize I was deficient in vitamin D until my bone doctor tested me for it. This vitamin is not included in a regular CBC and must be requested independently. Once I repaired my deficiency with supplements and lots of time in the sun, I began feeling more energized. Vitamin D3 is very important for bone repair and intestinal absorption, among other things. It makes sense that a deficiency here would allow cancer to take hold. If nutrients aren't being assimilated (which happens in the intestines), then the immune system will become weakened.

I'm going to talk about a factor now that I think is much more controversial even than animal products in the diet. I expect to get criticism over this, and many people will probably be very angry at me for talking so candidly about such a touchy subject, but it's my own personal opinion.

It's about smoking.

I believe smoking is a factor for cancer as much as anything else I've just mentioned. It's a stronger factor for some, than others, especially based on how much they smoke, and where in the body they happen to be weak. For me, smoking was just one of the myriad of factors that contributed to my cancer. I smoked for thirty years before I was finally able to quit and I totally believe it's a contributing factor for some, and a trigger for others. Just like a huge radiation dose might give one person cancer, but not another who was exposed in the same way, for the same amount of time, smoking is just another factor. Some people who never smoked a day in their life get lung cancer. Some people who've smoked nearly their entire life won't get lung cancer, or any type of cancer. The huge campaign against smoking has great intentions. It's brought a lot of awareness to the health hazards of smoking, and probably caused a great many people to quit. That's a wonderful thing! Maybe we should do it with everything that contributes to cancer; all the factors I've listed above, and then some; as long as someone's rights aren't being trampled on and they're not being ridiculed for their choices, awareness of anything dangerous is a good thing.

I think a person has to smoke an exorbitant amount in order for it to be a cancer trigger. With that said, I think any factor in abundance can possibly trigger cancer. Like that ER doctor said to me, "everyone has stress." Yes, everyone does have stress. The difference is, not everyone has the same amount of stress, or reacts the same way to stress. It's the same with all the other factors. That's why I think cancer is such a personalized entity and the cure can be different for each of us. I do believe there are cure-all's to cancer, as well (like a particular antibiotic will kill all of a specific bacteria). Those cure-all's are controversial because they are not endorsed, or even believed valid by the Western medical community. I don't list chemotherapy as one of those, by any means.

The reason I've gone on such a tangent about the tobacco subject is because I've seen the backlash the anti-smoking campaign has done, being on the other side of it, and it has caused a sort of "lynching" mentality for some people. I'm sure I'll do my fair share of trampling on someone's pet peeve in here, but people who blame someone's behavior for their cancer is my pet peeve. I have seen people do this to smokers, no matter what kind of cancer they have, without any regard for the facts, or FACTORS in their own lives that may or may not, could or could not, give THEMSELVES cancer. There is no room for blaming others or ourselves for our disease. There is room, however, for identifying and changing the factors in our OWN lives to prevent or treat our own disease. There are a plethora of factors that cause cancer in all of our lives that we can change. We have to live by example, not by judgment.

I continued to smoke for years after my diagnosis. I'd

quit for a few months here, and a few months there, but it never usually lasted long. It's no different from someone who eats meat having to give it up for whatever reasons, or anyone else trying to break an unhealthy habit, for that matter.

I was able to quit smoking in early 2012 by using electronic cigarettes, and patches. Of course a lot of sheer determination was helpful, and I believe eliminating that factor and replacing it with a healthy one helped, though I started smoking again in 2014. In the meantime, I spend more money for the organic, additive-free cigarettes simply because they're better.

I don't know how much of a factor smoking is in with my own cancer. I've cured myself of two mets while actively smoking, and my pulmonologist said he couldn't tell I was a smoker by looking at my lungs, so it probably isn't a big factor for me. It just proves how very different we all are.

Aside from the few factors I listed above, there are hundreds of other factors surrounding us that we can't necessarily control, but are probably aware of. Such as the toxins in our very air, and the water we drink.

I had been a vegetarian for fourteen years before my diagnosis, and colorectal cancer was the one cancer I consciously believed I would never get! It was a meat eater's disease, after all!

Vegetarians get colorectal cancer, people who've lived in communes away from freeways, microwave ovens and cigarettes, get cancer. Health fanatics who look to be in perfect physical condition get cancer. Babies get cancer. NO one is immune, and if they are, we have no idea who they are until they never get it. It's not until cancer shows up that we can try and look back to see what factors may have helped play a part. It usually takes years for cancer to show up, and by then, whatever may have triggered it would be far from our memories.

The radiation in our atmosphere is an unavoidable factor that has grown increasingly worse over the last several decades. Since before WWII, there have been innumerable nuclear detonations for testing, and for war, all over the world. The Chernobyl nuclear disaster by itself put megatons of radiation into the atmosphere that is still doing damage to us to this day.

This brings me to the next factor; genetics.

I am not a biologist or geneticist. This is just my opinion from observation and research. I believe that genes are usually a factor, and are not necessarily a trigger.

Why do some family members with a genetic disposition to cancer get it, and other family members who also have the gene do not? I think it's because of a trigger. Even FAP (Familial Adenomatous Polyposis), which supposedly has a 100% chance of occurring to the person who has the gene, could still be activated by a trigger. FAP causes multiple, sometimes thousands, of little adeno polyps to form on the large intestine, which will eventually become cancer if they're not removed. What appears to be happening is that doctors are removing the entire colon of people diagnosed with this gene before the gene is ever activated. It's a drastic preventative measure. I don't know the basis of their (the scientists) 100% statistic that everyone with the FAP gene will get cancer, but I've seen that number get tossed around by scientists before with a cancer that had a 100% mortality rate, and low and behold, someone survived it.

For anyone with FAP, all I can offer is my greatest support in whatever decision you choose. Just please do all the research you can, including using the resources I've listed in the appendix to get expert opinions on what can be done in a FAP, or any other gene specific situation and search out others who have it. There may possibly be a way to keep the gene from triggering, or to turn it off if it's already on.

Stress is probably the most common trigger for cancer. As I mentioned before, the doctor who treated my urinary blockage didn't buy that, but these days, even doctors are beginning to acknowledge the detriments of a stressful lifestyle.

The stress that triggered my cancer was prolonged and heavy. Maybe for others that much is not required. I have talked to many people who share this belief about their own cancer. A woman who developed breast cancer soon after her sister's death because she blamed herself for the tragedy, swore it was the stress that triggered it. All the factors in our lives have us ripe for a trigger, and what better trigger than a body that is being constantly under siege with worry and fear?

Many people I've talked to can correlate the beginning of their disease with some immensely stressful event. As I mentioned, few people realize this correlation because cancer usually takes years to develop before it's found, and by that time, the tragic event may have healed over or just too much time had passed for there to be a mental connection to the event/s. My tumor was 3-5 years old when it was found. By then, my mind and heart had mostly moved on from the cancer-causing event (divorce). As soon as the doctor aged my tumor that first week of diagnosis, I knew what triggered my cancer like a ton of bricks had fallen on my head. I think that was because I'd had such an immediate reaction to the stress, and because I became symptomatic nearly immediately afterwards.

I had most of the factors listed above, but I know without that life altering, eventful stress, it would've been many more years before cancer showed up in my body, if ever at all. And it may have eventually, with the factors I had, especially if I hadn't changed them somewhere along the line.

Environmental factors are the ones we can't really avoid. It's hardly worth mentioning these because there isn't much we can do about them short of moving to an island where there are no cars, or radio waves, or anything else we as a species release into the environment and even then, we're still bombarded by radiation from our atmosphere.

We may be able to reduce some of these environmental factors, though, depending on where on the planet we live and in what ways we can afford to change them.

Powerlines emit high frequency energy. It can be felt and heard just by being near them. Unfortunately, they're everywhere!

Carbon dioxide/monoxide. I know people who refuse to drive on the freeway with the windows rolled down. They believe keeping the windows up reduces the toxic carbon dioxide from the freeway entering the car. To me there is an even better possibility that keeping the windows rolled up traps the carbon dioxide from your own car in with you. I would just recommend not living near a freeway, or any other heavily trafficked road.

Off gases are another factor. These are usually from

items made of plastics and can sometimes smell awful. Any new plastic should be washed well with soap and water. Maybe give the item several washings if need be. Buy plastics that have no PCB's in them. Try not to breathe the smelly gases at all. They can come from new appliances, mattresses, and other items, too. Let those large items air out for at least 24 hours before use.

Some other small things we can do to limit our factors is to use more natural cleaning products and organic soaps and lotions. Stop using aerosol products such as hair sprays and insecticides, and basically live as chemical-free as possible.

I've come to believe hydrogen-peroxide (H2O2) is a miracle substance. One of its many uses is as a cleaning agent for counter tops, toilets, glass and teeth cleaning. It can even get some stains out of clothing, and works great in the laundry. Hydrogen-peroxide is even believed by some to cure cancer and there are doctors in the United States using it as a therapy.

My pulmonologist said my lungs were beautiful, even after a 30 year jaunt with cigarettes. I wasn't a heavy smoker, and I didn't breathe the smoke in very deeply. Maybe that's why I didn't get lung cancer instead of colorectal? Maybe the person who lived by powerlines his whole life got cancer because he had one, or four other factors that his sister didn't have so he got the cancer, and she didn't? Maybe a childhood trauma was never resolved and the emotions it caused kept the body in a constant state of stress, lowering the immune system until cancer eventually took hold? Maybe the immune system is simply weaker in one person, than another?

The possibilities are endless and only we as individuals

can trace back our recipe. By eliminating factors and annihilating the trigger, we can send cancer on the run. Even if the trigger is never identified, a person can still heal themselves by eliminating factors and by using the other methods I used that are listed in the next several chapters.

8.
TO EAT, OR NOT TO EAT

Okay, now it's time to have some fun and talk about my favorite subject!

Food!

Who doesn't like it, right?

I know people exist who don't care much for food, but I'm not one of them!

In fact, food and I have an extensive history that isn't all positive.

Anorexic/bulimic as a teenager, I starved myself for many months, and for many reasons. I was a street kid, so eating wasn't always a typical occurrence. It was more about not having food, than being afraid of becoming overweight. It wasn't long, though, before I realized what an easy tool starving myself was to control my weight.

Later on, just after my teenage years, the opposite started happening.

By the time I was 25, I was at least 50 lb. overweight.

I can't entirely blame food. Exercise was never a forte of mine and my lifestyle was very sedentary. Couple that with having a love for ANY kind of food, and it's the perfect recipe for being overweight.

I gave up meat when I was 25, but I was a junk food vegetarian for the most part.

Working and being a full time student made it even more challenging to control my weight and my eating habits were just terrible. I switched between junky food,

99

and healthy food, and before long I was nearly 100 lbs. overweight.

During my marital separation I started losing weight steadily. I walked regularly, and cut the fat out of my diet. Within a year, I lost sixty pounds.

By the time I was able to move out of my ex-husband's house, I was still very overweight, but a lot more confident to leave the house and participate in life again.

Over the next two years, my weight fluctuated between gaining and losing 25 lbs. I didn't understand why until I realized I had cancer. As I got sicker I wasn't able to eat as much, but wasn't losing as much weight. My diet had improved, but still wasn't the best in the world.

During the six month adjuvant chemo in 2008, I gained 74 lbs.! That was an average weight gain of 12 pounds per month! It was a combination of the steroids they were giving me for nausea, and not being at all careful about what I ate, or how much of it I ate. I felt horribly sick so much of the time, I totally justified eating a quart of Baskin Robbins peanut butter ice cream all in one or two sittings! That was something that I never used to allow myself to do.

After the ileostomy reversal, the exact opposite happened.

Eating became scary because nothing could pass the stricture. Everything I ate became a problem. I was spending so much of my life in the bathroom it was just like it was before the diagnosis. In some instances, it was even worse than before.

As I wrote in an earlier chapter, I went in for dilations every couple of months or so, but it never helped. All it would do was cause bowel incontinence for several days, then after that, nothing could pass through again.

It's taken years for me to figure food out and the first thing I discovered on the road to fixing the problem was probiotics, or the "good" bowel bacteria I talked about earlier.

It first came to me in the form of Kefir, a cultured yogurt drink available in just about any grocery store.

It took twelve hours for me to notice it was helping. Instead of having liquid stools, they were well formed, and almost felt normal. It was a HUGE change from what I'd been experiencing, and it was wonderful!

At that time, I had been reading many books on cancer, and non-Western ways of treating it. The information out there was not new, but it was NOT mainstream either.

Our bowels need a healthy amount of good bacteria to balance out the bad bacteria, and the medical doctors and self- educated nutritionists who wrote these books all new it. It was imperatively important.

My first question after my discovery of probiotics was why the hell hadn't the GI doctor told me about them? He's the bowel expert, and I had given him plenty of opportunities to tell me through my desperate questioning, but he never said a single word about them. None of the doctors did. Surely they knew about probiotics, didn't they?

Several of the books I had been reading talked about the healthcare industry, and the politics involved. Apparently doctors could only talk to patients about things they were taught in medical school, and could only prescribe things that had been FDA approved. Doctors receive very little to no educational training in nutrition in order to get their medical degree. They aren't given any tools about diet and its role in curing, or preventing illness, however, a doctor who believes probiotics could help a patient could be risking his medical license by recommending them. My first oncologist told me he had a patient die from taking probiotics which absolutely shocked me. To this day I have no idea why he would say such a thing, and I don't believe what he said was true.

Things have changed a lot since that time. Pharmaceutical companies have found ways to patent probiotic formulas and for the first time in the many years I've been dealing with doctors, my primary doctor, who knew nothing of my background at the time, recommended and prescribed me probiotics!

I'm glad the healthcare industry is beginning to understand the correlation between nutrition and illness, but as far as eating for a cure goes it is still only stragler doctors brave enough to stray away from the herd who are promoting nutrition as medicine. It's up to us as individual working parts of society who have to step up and start taking responsibility for our own health. We can't completely rely on the doctors to do it for us for several reasons. First of all, and I've said this before, we know our own bodies better than the doctors ever will. Secondly, doctors are under the controls of their licensing. The protocols that I believe are imperative to the cancer cure for all of us cannot be copyrighted, patented, or sold in any single combination. This is true because we are all so very different from each other, and so far, cancer has not been proven to be a virus, a bacteria, or any other organism that can be universally treated with pharmaceutical medicines. The fact that we're all different is something most mainstream doctors do not really seem to take into account when dealing with us. And they don't have much choice otherwise if we can't communicate our needs to them. First we must know our needs and sift through the choices of doctors until we find one that will listen to us as credible informants of our own bodies.

Of course there is a lot of controversy about what exactly proper nutrition is, and even amongst nutritionists, this topic can be, and often is, debatable.

From my own extensive research, I believe that proper nutrition is diverse, but a basic formula of a plant based diet is where all should start. From there, the modifications become VERY personalized. Ultimately, a person must do a lot of trial and error to customize what is healthy for them. Especially someone whose body has been cut up to the point of missing certain body parts essential for proper digestion! An illness compromises the immune system, and figuring out how to strengthen the immune system is ultimately important for proper health.

Finding what the perfect diet is for us individually is both the foundation and the pathway to healing for several reasons. First of all, and most importantly, is the way it makes us feel.

We MUST feel good and energized inside to heal from anything, and we can't feel as good as we need to with an unhealthy diet. This might be controversial to some until they actually experience what good nutrition can feel like. In healing, for me, the depression, the stress, the sluggishness, the sleeplessness, the pain...All of those feelings had to be conquered, and finding the perfect immune strengthening diet was the first step in doing that.

Being an ethical vegetarian for as many years as I was, it was a very challenging decision to start eating fish again.

103

The reason I did it was because my body was telling me to. I had a friend tell me years earlier that being an O blood type meant I needed more animal protein in my diet than some of the other blood types. I knew I was a type O, but my education, after working a vegetarian information booth for many years, was that eating meat and dairy was more protein than humans needed and that I could get all the protein I needed from veggies. I've found that it isn't necessarily the amount of protein so much as the type of protein that's important for some of us and we don't all have the same protein needs.

I started craving fish some months after my last round of chemo in 2008. I figured I was lacking omega-3, since fish was one of the few sources of that, so I added flax oil and flax seeds to my diet, and I mean A LOT of it. Flax is a great source of omega-3, but it's also a different type of omega-3, of course.

Well, my fingernails and hair grew stronger and thicker than ever, but I still felt sluggish, and was still craving fish.

By the time I had moved in with my grandmother, I was eating very healthy since my bathroom issues had not improved to my expectations after the ileostomy reversal. I was juicing a lot, and eating home-cooked meals the majority of the time. I had lost over 100 lbs., and my body was communicating very well what it needed. So in 2011, I took the plunge into fish eating.

Tuna salad was the first thing I had. Instead of getting crampy and sick as I was expecting, my energy level increased, and my fatigue nearly disappeared over night.

Everything about my health began changing after that.

I figured out that too much fiber in my diet was not a good thing because fibrous waste couldn't easily get

104

passed the stricture. That limited my juicing, which also limited my nutrition. I started supplementing more with a multi-vitamin, vitamin D3, capsuled probiotics, calcium, chaga, and alkaline tablets. I was walking better, and soon developed some flexibility in my stiff, sedentary joints. The chronic tailbone fracture still caused problems, but I was learning my limitations with that; no bending or squatting.

I learned that rice was a great staple for me, and I discovered sushi! Never thought in my life I would want to eat that! I started with the cooked stuff, and very slowly moved into trying raw fish. Nothing in my diet made me feel more energetic and healthy than eating sushi. Seaweed is a miracle superfood to me. It is high in iodine, which is perfect for those of us who've had, and continue to have, radiation treatments and/or regular radiation doses from CT scans and x-rays. There are a myriad of different types of seaweeds. Nori and wakame are my favorites. Dulse comes in a shaker sometimes and can be used as a seasoning. The best place to get seaweed and other Asian specific foods is at an Asian market. Most major cities have them.

My diet is still a work in progress, and probably always will be. I gained weight when I stopped smoking and continued to struggle with it until recently.

Once I started realizing my personal nutritional needs, the rest started falling into place.

The Ayurvedic philosophy is one of my favorite ways of eating, too, as it incorporates all seven flavors essential for eliminating unhealthy cravings, and overall good health. I mix that up with limited gluten, limited refined sugar, and over all plant based eating, and feel I've really found what works best for me. Now, with everything I cook, I add the Ayurvedic philosophy with the seven flavors; spicy, salty, sweet, bitter, pungent, sour and astringent.

Mix up the experimentation with different and new kinds of foods. Find what tastes good that's healthy, and work with it. I always add what I need, and eliminate what doesn't make me feel good. A nutritious meal should create uplifting feelings with lots of energy. A non-nutritious meal will have us feeling lethargic, with a lack of energy, and possibly even running for the toilet. Eating too much can do that too, so be careful of that. I pay close attention to how my body reacts with certain foods, and I know my bowel clock. In other words, it takes me about 24 hours to digest most foods. People with faster metabolisms might digest in 12 hours. This is the best way to know what is working for you. Your bowel movement will tell you everything you need to know about that meal. Don't be afraid to look at it and remember if it was difficult to pass, liquid, or colorless, because those are not good signs. I kept a food journal for easy reference and added how my body reacted to whatever food I ate. I would continually try new foods, or foods that weren't normally eaten. I know from experience a person can develop a strong liking for a food that was previously loathed. When I first became a vegetarian, I hated all vegetables except broccoli. Now I love almost all of them.

I would start with either a vegan or raw diet for a month, and see how that feels. Then build from there, adding and eliminating foods as needed. Buy, or find online, several cookbooks about each interesting diet and read through them. Anything make your mouth water?

106

Just stay away from the meat cookbooks while doing this! It isn't worth the toxic effects, or the cancer and heart disease risks to eat it. If someone is eating to manage or rid themselves of disease, it's much better to stay away from animal products until you have a handle on the situation. It's my personal belief that the only meat humans are meant to eat are fish and insects, and most of us can do fine without even those. Someone once told me that she was confused about what to eat because everything seemed contaminated or poisoned. She's pretty much right. All we can do is the best we can do with our own research, and our own choices, but when eating for a cure, animal products are not good; even fish, unless raw.

If one finds themselves just too addicted to stop eating red meat, chicken or pork, then eat organic, farm raised animals, and in very limited quantities. This is for the long-term, though; as I just said, and I'll say it again and again and again, no animal products while eating to heal. These are things that should be gradually introduced back into the diet after we're well, or on "maintenance."

Organic juicing is probably the single most healthy task a person can add to their diet for overall good nutrition, and has been known to turn disease around. I have read several stories about people who have claimed to cure their cancer by adding this one simple task to their lifestyle, and doing it at least once a day, if not exclusively all day.

The Gerson Method uses heavy juicing in their program. They do it 13 times per day, and then have a healthy vegan dinner. I listed references for Gerson in the appendix. They have a very impressive survival rate.

Juicing definitely makes me feel supergized! I add

some pretty powerful supplements to my juice which sure adds a nutritional wallop to it. My favorite things to juice are carrots, kale, apples, lemons, beets, and blueberries. Sometimes I add celery, cucumber, strawberries, and dandelion. The supplements I add are powdered spirulina, MSM, bee pollen, maca, camu camu, and sometimes goji berry. I made a list in the next chapter of the cancer-fighting foods I know of. Many of which can be juiced. The stricture limits my juicing capabilities because of the liquid stool factor, so I try to eat a lot of whole, raw, fruits and veggies, and juice only occasionally.

The juicer I use is the Champion. It's recommended that persons with cancer (or any serious illness) use only masticating, or pressing juicers. The centrifugal ones destroy too much of the plant cell walls, causing faster oxidation of the juice, and faster break-down of the nutrients. I LOVE my Champion juicer! They're not cheap, but they're sold pre-owned for pretty reasonable prices on eBay. Just make sure you're buying from a reputable seller. The quality of the Champion is awesome. Even though mine is used, and looks old, it's been going strong since I bought it in 2009.

The best juicers on the market are the pressing juicers. There aren't many companies I know of that make these, and they're terribly expensive. But if the financial means are there, get one of these. They have both commercial and home models. A company I know that makes a great press juicer is "Green Star".

If a juicer is not an option, then a blender and cheesecloth will work just fine. Put all the ingredients (minus the hard seeds) into a blender, and then pour the mixture into a bowl or pitcher lined with cheesecloth.

Then simply strain all the liquid into the bowl through the cheesecloth. If you don't mind a really pulpy or frothy drink, don't worry about straining it. I use the pulp to either make garden burgers, or give it to Rainbow and my other pug that I adopted last year, Oliver.

Now a word on sugar.

Like protein, fats and carbs, all sugars are NOT created equal.

Many of the fruits and veggies I listed above for juicing contain a LOT of natural sugars. Just so happens, cancer LOVES sugar. In fact, the PET scan, which is a cancer detecting scan, works by seeing where there is an unusually high sugar consumption going on in the body. If there is an unnatural rate of sugar metabolism in a specific area, it's most likely cancer having a feeding frenzy on the radioactive glucose they inject, which is sugar. It amazes me that the doctors aren't telling their patients not to eat simple sugars, but here again it could be the limitations of their licensing.

The one thing about this revelation that's apparent to me is that natural sugars have health benefits that refined sugars completely lack. Beyond that, it's my personal belief that refined sugar is the devil and should be avoided as much as possible; completely avoided if eating to heal. This includes high fructose corn syrup, brown sugar, powdered sugar, and even some sugars that claim to be raw. I'm going to be a killjoy again and add breads, pasta and rice to that list. They become the same thing as refined sugar in the body. Instead, I use stevia, agave, bananas, applesauce, raw honey, and occasionally (rarely) palm sugar to sweeten things. Oh, wait until you try my apple bars recipe in the back of the book...Mmmm!!

Gluten is another food that is absolutely useless in our diets.

I mentioned gluten in a previous chapter, and now I'm going to rip it to shreds.

I don't know why we started using wheat in place of the ancient grains such as millet in our diet, but somehow, that mistake was made, much to our detriment.

The health dangers of gluten have become more mainstream in recent years as more people have discovered a marked difference in health by reducing gluten in the diet.

Some years ago, a colorectal cancer friend of mine mentioned that she was convinced gluten was the cause of colorectal cancer. I thought it was an interesting theory, so I experimented with it by eliminating it for a while, then slowly incorporating it back into my diet, then giving it up, and then eating a lot of it.

I noticed immediately a difference in how my body felt each time I gave gluten up for any period of time. The only way I can describe it is that I felt "lighter". Even more noticeably, my stricture felt less problematic. After more experimentation, I discovered that gluten causes inflammation inside my body, so that was why I felt lighter, and the stricture felt less swollen when I wasn't eating it.

It was convincing enough evidence for me.

I no longer cook with wheat products, and eat gluten only occasionally.

Cutting meat out of my diet was an ethical decision, having nothing to do with health. I always figured the health benefits were just a lucky bonus.

Unfortunately, I discovered very early on that just

because you don't eat meat, doesn't mean you're eating healthy!

The saying, "there's plenty to eat, without choosing meat", is the truest statement, ever!

Fried zucchini, French fries, quesadillas, enchiladas, potato chips with sour cream dip, pizza...I sure didn't suffer eating like a rabbit!

I gained a lot of weight being a vegetarian, as I've mentioned, and had absolutely no energy, all the time. I didn't like vegetables all that much, and had to teach myself how to love them in their true forms.

It's so strange to look back on those days.

I mentioned in a previous chapter that I believed colorectal cancer was the one cancer I was immune to because it was a meat-eaters disease. I know so many vegetarians who have this very cancer! It goes to show that knowledge is ever expanding and becoming outdated even as I write this.

I drink coffee rarely, if ever. Maybe once every six months. I did get in the habit of drinking soy chai latte tea, but decided it probably wasn't good for me from a coffee shop and gave it up.

My favorite thing to drink is ice water with lemon in it. I believe lemon has incredible health benefits and I put lemon on everything, rind and all! This is beneficial in both warm and iced water.

Another trick I occasionally do, or used to do a lot, was fast. It can be uncomfortable, but giving the intestinal tract a break once in a while is healthy. The fast, or cleanse I would do is called the Master Cleanse, or Lemonade diet is another name for it. There is an easy recipe for it online, but I adjust it to my personal taste. It's simply water, grade a, or b maple syrup, lemon juice, and powdered cayenne pepper. The fast can be done for up to 21 days, but I've never gone longer than eight days. The cleanse worked for me with weight loss and in getting relief from my strictures for several days. Now I only use it as my bowel prep for my colonoscopies. Because of the stricture, the poop juice doesn't guarantee a clean out for me anymore so I do a three to four day fast, instead. Sometimes it works, sometimes it doesn't.

Another kind of fasting is juice fasts which I've always wanted to do, but can't do completely because of the stricture. These can be done healthily for an indefinite amount of time. I would just use a wide variety of fruits and veggies, with lots of lemon. Both of these fasts are good for losing weight, too. If weight loss is something not wanted, juicing should not cause any significant weight loss. Being overweight isn't healthy so eating super healthy naturally causes the body to drop weight. Being underweight isn't any less unhealthy so a weight gain may be experienced when eating healthily. The experience will be everything balancing out.

I know the foods that are ultimately unhealthy for me, but I still eat them occasionally. Nothing at all wrong with that! I just try not to get carried away with it. I allow myself to have a bit of pizza layered with cheese about once every few months, or even less often than that, sometimes. I still once in a while have a piece of chocolate cake. By allowing myself these little pleasures, I'm staying healthy by staying happy. During the times I had cancer actively in my body, I stayed away from all the really bad items that were loaded with refined sugar. I always try to stay away from refined sugars, and make my own food the majority of the time.

I will add briefly because it's relevant here, that sometime in 2010, a new spot on my good lung lit up on a PET scan. As we prepared to do surgery on it, I began juicing heavily that entire next month. When a CT scan was done on it a month or so later, the spot had mysteriously vanished. My oncologist was visibly stunned, but said it could have been a misread, or something. He didn't sound convinced, and I wasn't, either. From what I've read, PET scans are fairly accurate and false/positives are not common. That is what I refer to as my unofficial recurrence. Even though I believe it was a recurrence that heavy juicing got rid of, since it was never biopsied, I have to admit that it could have been a fluke.

It was no fluke when in May of 2016, the colon met that had been lighting up the PET scans for nearly a year, suddenly disappeared without a trace after five weeks of eating nothing but raw food.

Is it possible that diet is the pathway that leads to the cure? Faced with the evidence, it's certainly a great place to start.

9.
SUPPLEMENTS, CHOW, AND HOW NOW?

I stopped supplementing in 2012, after my lobectomy. My body seems to no longer need them and the only things I take now are my probiotics.

Supplements can be very useful if a person is not able to eat as much as they should, or if they're deficient in something particular. Even then, they should only be used for a short period of time. When experimenting with a diet, it might be a good idea to supplement until there's no longer any need to.

I think everyone should have their D3 blood levels tested, especially if cancer is the diagnosis or if there is a high risk for getting cancer. I wrote earlier that it's my strong belief that a deficiency in this key vitamin is a factor in getting cancer. The D3 test is not included in a CBC, and must be specifically requested by a doctor. My osteo doctor requested it for me just before the tailbone fracture was found, and bone metastasis was suspected. Low and behold, I was deficient.

I began supplementing in high doses, and spending lots of time in the sun.

Taking supplements should always be done wisely, and conscientiously. It is possible to overdose on vitamins, and that can be dangerous.

While trying to bolster my D3 levels, I was taking about 10,000 iu's per day, and spending hours in the sun. I did this for a year. I got D3 toxicity which was horrible abdominal cramps, and headaches. Took me a while to figure this out, especially with everything else that was going on in my body!

I took high levels of D3 after my deficiency diagnosis, but I did it for too long. A normal, safe amount to take is around 1500 iu's per day. My multi-vitamin also had some D3 in it, so that added to taking too much. Be careful when taking supplements and don't go over the recommended daily dose unless a specialist has told you otherwise. I will list the companies I prefer for each supplement in the appendix.

Another great discovery for me, and a great recommendation from my friend Aaron, was Chaga.

Chaga is a bark-like mushroom that grows on birch trees. It is used a lot in Chinese medicine, and is referred to as the "King of Herbs" in China. It is a known cancer killer, as many mushrooms are.

I supplemented Chaga in capsule form for about a year, and although I don't know if it helped me at all (I took it too sporadically), if chaga can be obtained in a tea form, I think people with cancer should take it like that. I got it from my traditional Chinese doctor. I eat as many different kinds of mushrooms as I can get, as often as I can, cooked. Maitake mushrooms are another type that have powerful cancer fighting properties, but so do Reiki and Shiitake. I've heard negative things about button, white, crimini or portabella mushrooms, which I think some of those are the same species, but I've never had a problem eating them. I mostly just use the Asian mushrooms.

More on Probiotics: They can be supplemented, or found in drinks, yogurt and certain foods. I've mentioned probiotics several times before, and believe they are crucial for colorectal cancer people. As far as supplementing with capsules…it works okay for me, but I still prefer getting it from my food and drinks. They should be taken on an empty stomach. Some experts recommend taking a probiotic supplement with 12 different probiotic strains. Some of the drinks and foods that have probiotics in them won't list the strains, or amounts of strains, but that's okay. A supplement along with eating and drinking fermented foods works for me, and probably will for most people. As far as getting probiotics in foods, you can't overdose. Sour Kraut or Kimchi is the best food sources I can think of. I take two capsules per day, and drink 8 oz. of Kombucha per day, every day, if I can.

I've tried nearly every kind of probiotic, and most work to some extent or other. I have a brand I think is the best on the market. I will include them in the supplement list, and also where to get great deals on them.

"Kombucha", which is a highly fermented tea, has both a bitter and sour taste, and is fizzy. Some people find it unpalatable and it may take some getting used to, but I am still experimenting with different flavors and companies. Rejuvelac is another highly fermented drink loaded with probiotics that I've tried. It's not my favorite, but if you seriously want to get probiot-icked, that is the drink for you!

Miso is fermented soy beans. It's an item that is inexpensive at Asian markets, but also available at most health food stores for a price. It comes in a variety of styles; red, white and yellow. I prefer yellow because it's mild, but not too mild. I mostly use it in soup bases.

As far as trace minerals go, be careful when supplementing these. There is strong evidence that we're overdosing on them.

We should only be getting small amounts of these. Trace minerals include iron, zinc, and copper which are considered heavy metals. We get these and other trace elements not just from our food, but from our pots and pans. I lightly mentioned earlier that aluminum was a cancer factor. Well, most pots and pans on the market these days are made of aluminum. I've also eliminated cast iron and copper pots and pans from my cookware items because the minerals may leech into the food. Stainless steel, so far, is safest to cook with.

I will always believe that getting proper nutrition should be relied upon with food rather than with supplements, but for some, it's challenging to eat enough to get proper nutrition and for others, proper absorption can be the real culprit. Those of us with any kind of digestive cancer might have an absorption issue.

Enzymes are the catalysts of life. Without them, life ceases to happen.

Being a biology major, I always knew this. I don't know why it took me so long to figure out that I needed to add enzymes to my diet before anything else. Even before the probiotics I should've been taking pancreatic enzymes!

They were the final piece of my nutritional puzzle in the beginning.

The enzymes I added are probably the reason why my body eliminated the need to take the other supplements.

For a while I suspected that I wasn't properly absorbing nutrients. I feared that my pancreas wasn't doing its job right, and after being diagnosed with diabetes in 2009 after the six month weight gain, malabsorption was probably a lot of what was going on.

An indication of malabsorption can be found in the stool. When in fear, check your rear. The stools were greasy, full of mucous, and very pale. This could've meant several things, but the one that made sense for me was that I wasn't getting nutrients.

Again, everything changed when I added enzymes to my diet.

It started with an article I found in my research about something or other.
It was from the U.K., and it was explaining the importance of enzymes in the fight against cancer.

The article, published by anticancerinfo.co.uk, educates the reader on the vitamin B17 in particular. B17, or nitrilosides, is found in millet, apricot kernels, and apple seeds. I found the article most interesting, and most credible for many reasons. First of all, the study was done by Krebs, et al, who science majors all know as Dr. Ernst Krebs, discoverer of the Krebs cycle, the cycle in which cells convert food into energy. Krebs, et al, discovered that cancer cells all have a protective protein barrier around them that make them impenetrable from the body's natural defenses and other things that would otherwise kill them. If the protein barrier could be dissolved, the cancer cells would become vulnerable enough to easily be destroyed. The enzymes they found that dissolved the protein barrier were trypsin and a-chymotrypsin. The formula they recommend that seems to have the highest concentration of both enzymes, is called Univase Forte.

I started taking it in late 2012, and I believe it aided in

my overall nutritional health. It also made my hair thick!

As wheat replaced millet in our diets, so was a great, natural cancer killer. Millet, and ancient grain, has very high cancer-fighting abilities. I now do most of my baking with millet flour.

Here is my grocery list for cancer-less foods, and some of the foods that will be included in the cancer-esa-peas chapter. All items should preferably be organic, but asterisk items should definitely be organic;

Broccoli*

Lemon

Turmeric

Millet (flour, and otherwise)

Apples*

Avocados

Garlic

Zucchini*

Maitake Mushrooms*

Shitake Mushrooms*

Crimini Mushrooms*

Mushrooms

Alfalfa Sprouts*

(wild caught)   Quince

Coconut oil

Brocolli Sprouts*

Carrots*

Kale*

Seaweed (nori, wakame, dulce)

Chili Peppers

Red Grapes*

Apricot Kernels

Oranges

Grapefruit

Bamboo Shoots

Raspberries*

Buckwheat

Cassava

Barley

Brown Rice

Blackberries*

Reishi

Smoked Salmon

Cinnamon

Raw Honey *

Stevia (sweetener)

Bananas

Beets

Pomegranite

Blueberries*   Miso
Tomatoes*
Nuts
Flaxseed/oil
Soy (non-GMO, if possible)
Green and Black Tea
Figs
Rosemary
Spinach*
Beans
Cabbage*
Cauliflower*
Sweet Potatoes
Fenugreek Tea
Unsweetened Applesauce

The blank spaces in the list can be used to add other foods that I haven't mentioned to the cancer-less list. There are many more, and new ones are always being discovered.

I believe a diet rich in variety is optimum. There are a few items I try to eat with everything, like turmeric, cinnamon, and lemon, but eating a high variety of fruits and vegetables ensures I'm getting proper nutrition.

There is a controversy about B17 in apricot kernels, that when ingested it releases cyanide into the body causing cyanide poisoning. The only foods listed above that have this potential danger are the apricot kernels, and apple seeds. I have been taking apricot kernels intermittently since 2009, and have had no problems with it at all. The most I take at one time is ten kernels. I've never heard of anyone having a problem taking these, but of course, if you're allergic, don't eat them at all. The flip side to this controversy by the supporters of laetrile (apricot kernels) in curing cancer is that the medical industry is trying to scare people against taking laetrile because it really is the cure! There is plenty of information floating around out there about it, so all I can say is research it and make an educated decision before taking it, or anything else.

Another word on enzymes.

There are natural ways besides supplementing to promote natural enzyme production. Fenugreek tea is a wonderful item to add to the diet. It has many health benefits, including possibly stimulating the body's natural production of pancreatic enzymes.

10.
Get Yer Degree On;
Ph. D N. ME

Just like there are a myriad of ways to get cancer, there are probably even more ways of curing it. To know and understand that cancer is VERY curable is the perfect attitude to have. It's my strongest belief that the human body is not only capable of, but very well designed to repair, regenerate, and thrive from illness and injury. If the injury or illness doesn't kill you instantly, you CAN survive it, no matter what it is. Our body wants to be healthy. It wants to live, and it will work with us to achieve this. It only needs our assistance.

Many of us have heard of seemingly miraculous healings...the child who lived for years without a brain, the man who survived an arrow straight through his noggin, or the woman who jumped out of an airplane from 10,000 feet, and hit the ground after her parachute failed. She broke every bone in her body, but she lived. These people survived the un-survivable. Whether you believe those are miracles, or not, it shows that anything is possible with the human body and spirit.

There is no reason why those healings can occur, and ours can't. No matter what stage of disease we're currently in. No matter what degree of what stage the illness is in, the body CAN heal. Millions of years of evolution have perfected our defense mechanisms against foreign bodies, including the ones that aren't so foreign; like cancer.

In my research, I came across so much wonderful and useful information that helped me in learning how to listen to, and communicate with my own body. Dr. Weil's book, Spontaneous Healing, helped me immensely in figuring out my diet. I recommend that anyone facing a major healing challenge, or anyone who wants to improve their overall health and well-being, simply read as much as they can about other people's experiences and subjects on natural healing. Even though doctors are not by their training nutritionists and receive very little education on that front, many have gone out on their own and become experts in the field. Coupled with their medical training, some of them have developed some pretty provocative information regarding food as medicine. Besides Dr. Weil, I recommend reading anything by Dr. Neal Barnard from PCRM.org.

I immersed myself in all the information I could get on the subject. There was plenty of information out there by the medical community telling me my odds of surviving my type of cancer and stage were next to impossible, and I didn't want to believe that. I couldn't believe that. Ultimately, I didn't believe that.

All the books I chose to read told me instead that I could live and beat my disease. That I could heal myself and that was all I needed to get me started. Actually, the thing that got me started was a woman I met on the CSN website. I'll call her Valerie E.

She had been cancer-free for several years already when I first met her, but her story didn't start off that way.

After years of ineffective treatments and many recurrences, she came to a place in her disease where she was no longer "treatable." There were multiple tumors in her lungs and liver, and no known chemotherapy or mixture therein was working. Her doctors sent her home, regrettably with the expectation she wouldn't live but the next few months.

Valerie E. did go home, but she didn't die within the next few months. She began juicing organic fruits and vegetables, did master cleanses, and completely changed her lifestyle to one promoting a cancer-free body.

She went into non-surgical remission, with every tumor vanishing. To this day, some ten plus years later, she remains cancer-free.

That was my first real-life experience with someone who knew she could, and did. Her story was the most inspiring in my life, and in my decision to go it naturally and take responsibility for my own health.

I don't know exactly everything Valerie E. did to cure herself aside from the things I listed, but I soon learned that it didn't entirely matter what she herself did. What was important was what I was doing, and that was finding my own way. I found that diet was an important factor, but in the beginning, it was only 2/10th's of the cure, for me. Like I've stated earlier, it took me a long while to realize, nutrition was the pathway. I still needed to get rid of my cancer-trigger. Two other ingredients proved to be the actual building blocks, and ultimately the most important in my healing. I have no idea if these same factors played a part in Valerie E.'s cure, but I suspect some of it did.

Once I learned it could be done, that it had been done,

the floodgates were open, and my insatiable desire for knowledge about self-healing was unleashed.

The book I most recommend for individuals dealing with cancer is "Anticancer, A New Way of Life", by David Servan-Schreiber, MD, Ph.D. This book was written by a medical doctor who got brain cancer and not only refused his prognosis, but his doctor's recommended treatment. As a result, he survived twenty years passed the expiration date they gave him and wrote that very informative, very important book.

Dr. Servan-Schreiber's story proves that we can heal ourselves of a difficult-to-survive cancer without deadly chemicals that promote disease rather than cure it.

How well do we know our own bodies? Better than anyone else. Better even than our doctors. No matter how much education someone has, they cannot know our body better than us. It isn't possible. When we're sick, getting in touch with our own bodies is so very important. If we don't know our own bodies very well, it just makes it that much harder for our doctors to understand them. If we can tell our doctors precisely what our bodies are telling us, and if the doctors listen, we can work in better conjunction together, and healing will be that much easier. Doctors who diagnose us based on other cases they have seen, or based on their own intuition are going to hit it wrong a lot. On the same hand, it is our responsibility to learn how to communicate our symptoms to our doctors, and strongly advocate for what we believe we need. It's not our responsibility to become a medical doctor, but I truly believe it is our responsibility to become an expert on our own bodies. Of course it is! There is no other way we can live in excellent health and excellent vitality without being in close mental contact with our own physical body. We are all educated in our own bodies to an extent, and though another person can help guide us along the path of learning about ourselves, ultimately, only we can know ourselves.

I hold a Ph.D. N. ME, which simply means I am an expert on my own body. I may not know the exact function of every system, but no expert can know every single minute detail about their subject.

Occasionally I would ask my good friend who holds a Ph.D. in organic chemistry a question about some organic substance or other, and every time he would tell me he didn't know.

"You don't know?" I would say, stunned. "Aren't you an expert in this field?" By which he would respond, "The subject is too broad for anyone to know everything about it."

It's the same with our own bodies. Just because we don't know the Kreb cycle, or the processes in which nutrients are absorbed by the small intestines, doesn't mean we're not experts on our own bodies. Our body and cells are intelligent and communicate with us all the time. At least they try to. The language they speak isn't verbal, so it's up to us to learn how to decipher what they're saying.

Western medicine is based entirely on subjects that produce results in a lab or study. Even then, it isn't considered a fact, or law, until it repeats the same result several times over. Life simply has more components than "science" can understand or explain; our bodies being the best example of that.

Dr. Gabriel Cousens, in his book, The Rainbow Diet,

talks about studies done in labs in which rats were given a particular substance, and when the urine of the rats was tested, somehow, their bodies had produced more molecules of the substance than they had been given. Somehow, the rat's bodies created molecules that didn't exist before.

That study goes against everything science has proved true in the law of thermodynamics. In other words, it was an impossibility according to science, yet, it happened. Science cannot explain everything and therefore cannot be relied upon for everything.

Our bodies are a Universe within themselves. Combined, yet separate from the Universe outside of us.

Just look at it. Imagine what it takes for our bodies to function, to live, to exist. It doesn't take a science major to realize it takes a lot of team work for our bodies to function properly. It's amazing to think about how much can go wrong between one function and the next, yet usually, amazingly, nothing major goes wrong enough to kill us. Usually, the systems of the body do their jobs properly, and can easily fix any little thing that might go wrong from time to time.

If something major does go wrong, our body tries to alert us to this in the form of symptoms. Many people will say they experienced no symptoms from their disease. Symptoms can be very subtle, and they don't always express themselves in the same ways for everyone. Sometimes all we have to do is communicate with our bodies once in a while to keep on par with our body's needs and complaints, and then finding problems or illness becomes easier.

11.

BELIEF IS 4/10th's OF THE LAW

The second step in my formula for curing my cancer is as simple as it sounds, and goes back to the introduction. BELIEVING I CAN cure it, and changing my conditioned emotional responses to it, as well as my conditioned emotional responses to everything else in my life.

It's my belief that the human mind is the most powerful thing in existence. It's where our most amazing superpowers are located. In our collective Universe (the one we're all in together), and in our individual Universe (our own bodies), we are the masters. This may seem like an anti-God ideology, but it really isn't. If God is inside us, that makes him/her part of us. There are probably a hundred different ways to look at the theory without destroying the belief systems of anyone. Without getting to theological, let's just stick with the idea that the mind is very powerful.

There is certainly plenty of evidence to suggest that our minds can control our bodily functions as well as other things in our environment. I know from experience that such things are very real. In most of my own research, I've spent countless hours being my own guinea pig, and yes, psychosomatics is most certainly a real phenomenon. I have triggered abdominal cramping and bathroom issues on dozens of occasions just by thinking about it inadvertently. When it was at its highest annoyance, all I had to do was think about eating something and the bathroom issues would start full board. I learned eventually to be very conscientious of my thoughts, and in doing so, I was slowly able to control my bathroom problems to an extent. I could at least stop the issues when I realized they were being triggered by my thoughts. When the heavy cramping starts up, I stop what I'm doing, and concentrate on relaxing the area where the pain is. I focus completely on calming that area, and the pain sometimes will subside. Learning relaxation techniques can greatly increase your control over your symptoms, and this is a form of psychosomatics.

Watching how Rainbow recovered from her own cancerous tumor surgery has also taught me a lot about psychosomatics.

A day after having a wide incision tissue removal from her chest and armpit, she barely limped that first day. The day after that, she was walking around normally, and seemed to barely have any pain. Then the day after that was a perfectly normal day, aside from some itching, she acted as if nothing had ever happened. She didn't know what had been done to her, so she didn't have any of the mental stuff telling her she'd been through a physically traumatic event that should incapacitate her for weeks or that should cause her a ton of pain. Most importantly, she didn't have the mental imagery of being sliced open and torn apart, which gives those of us who know better the major creepies.

Scientists have been using psychosomatics in studies for years. When a placebo is given to a person participating in a study and they're told it's the medicine that will help them, there are usually some participants in the study for whom the placebo works. This was the person's own belief system healing them. Being the masters of their own Universe, they created the event (self-healing), without even knowing it. We can achieve the same success when we know about it, too.

A cancer diagnosis for most people is a horrible, shocking experience. All the blood leaves the head, and it feels like a judge just handed down a death sentence.

I didn't experience that feeling upon my first diagnosis. As I said earlier, I was relieved beyond imagination that they were able to diagnose me at all. I also had the luxury of knowing within myself before-hand, that it was most likely cancer, regardless that everyone else thought otherwise. I did, however, have that sheer feeling of dread after I discovered I had metastasis. I felt the grief; I felt the strong sense of loss. I felt all the classic feelings people report feeling. I let myself feel the fear and grief for the remainder of that first day. The next day, I completely flipped over my attitude about it.

I sat down in front of my computer, and I researched everything I could on alternative treatments, and most importantly, I sought out people who had defeated a stage IV colorectal cancer diagnosis and got motivation and inspiration from them. I created a plan of action for myself. I plotted a day by day itinerary of what I was going to do to improve my health, and my life. I didn't do it with a feeling of desperation. I felt motivated, and inspired. I never let the thought of dying interfere with my plans. It wasn't an option. After that first day, I never let myself believe I was going to die of the disease. Not today, not tomorrow, and not in forty years. It was more than a belief. It was a fact I knew inside myself, because that's what I wanted to believe. Whether or not I was fooling myself didn't matter, and it still doesn't matter. If there was a way for me to survive, I was going to find it, and I have. I refuse to live by a bucket list, but I definitely live to enjoy my life.

I didn't let anyone tell me I couldn't do it, and wow, were there people telling me I couldn't do it! The first oncologist never said it, but the look on his face each time he saw me told me how he felt about it. And he continually tried to get me to do chemo. Even the new oncologist, who was into more natural treatment options was insisting I do chemo, at first. The oncologist did tell me that chemo was my best chance for survival, and he may have believed that, but I certainly didn't.

I had done too much research and had too much information to trust that chemo was the cure for me. I trusted my body. I BELIEVED in my body, and I knew in my gut that I was stronger than the cancer.

Even when I got my second recurrence, where the tumor in my lung was doing triple time growth and I felt the fear for a longer period of time, I continued implementing my plan, and stayed pretty focused on it. Despite all the hoops I had to jump through to get the surgery, and having to see all new doctors, I was a seasoned veteran by then and the stress motivated me instead of breaking me down. It's how I know I'm going to survive many years longer than is typical for this disease and stage, and may eventually be free of it forever.

To believe something so strongly that you know it's a fact is the act of creating your own Universe. We all have this superpower. It just needs perfected and strengthened through practice and determination. Once I started seeing the results of my beliefs, they only grew more real and my resolve and determination grew ever stronger. I have the confidence to know I can live through ANYTHING that doesn't immediately kill me. I have the confidence to know I can accomplish ANYTHING I put my mind to. It's MY choice, and I'm in control of how I feel, as well as how I heal.

Some people have this strong of a belief in God. For them, prayer works, and many have experienced "miracles" through the act of group prayer. If this was in fact God answering the prayer because enough people asked for it, or whether the power of belief willed the miracle to happen, is definitely up for interpretation. I believe that both are possible.

The power of prayer is something I believe in full heartedly. Even though I am not a theologically religious person, I am deeply spiritual. I believe when we combine the power of our beliefs as a communal force and concentrate our energy on something together, we can accomplish any miracle we put our minds to whether it's reaching out to a God, or creating the event with our own minds. One of the most wonderful things about life is the possibilities it holds. Combining our superpowers to work together is how we create and change our shared Universe, be it mentally, or physically.

Possibilities are everywhere we look, and for anything we desire. I often close my eyes and imagine my inner Universe without cancer. I do that continually, and often. I experience the feeling of being healthy, and hold onto it. It's real.

There are many environments in which cancer can thrive. A healthy, happy, body and mind, is NOT one of them. I accept the challenge cancer has bestowed on me to BELIEVE myself cancer-free. I'm the only one who can do it.

12.
LOOKING FOR THE CURE;
Finding the Purpose

I've heard other cancer survivors talking about how cancer has been a gift or a blessing in their lives. I've even heard survivors tell a story of how cancer was the best thing that ever happened to them.

Cancer means different things to different people, of course. I've seen different aspects of its effects, both positive, and negative. I've seen those who get angry with the disease and hate it, and for some, that attitude never changes to the day they die. I've seen those who have the most positive attitudes about their disease, and that never seems to change until the day they die, either. I've also seen people with both attitudes defeat it.

Why do some people survive while others don't? It's the second biggest cancer question many of us have. I gave my own theories in a previous chapter. All I know for certain is how and why I got mine and how I figured out the best way for ME to deal with it.

Finding purpose in my disease, finding purpose in myself, finding purpose in my life and in everything having to do with my life, helped my belief that I acquired my disease for a reason. Once I figured out what that reason was, I changed it, and put a big chink in cancer's plan for me.

I know what I myself have experienced, and I always

knew I was going to survive my disease. Yes, we all have to die of something, someday, but at 47 years of age, that time, for me, wasn't, and isn't now. It wasn't at 38, either.

I believe that those of us who die from this disease, or of any torturous illness, do so because we eventually choose to. Myself having been in the position where giving into death felt more like a luxury, I understand very well about giving up. Fighting a painful illness is exhausting by every stretch of the imagination. I often fantasized about the relief death would bring, and about being somewhere else, far away from my suffering body. Every night while I struggled for comfort, I wished for death. When there's no light at the end of the tunnel, how can anyone blame someone for letting go? I believe each one of us who lingers knows when to let go, even if we don't really want to. I fully believe it's a choice. I'm by no means saying that those of us who keep getting recurrences are getting them because we want to die. That isn't the case, at all. My recurrences were my body's way of telling me I wasn't fixing what was wrong. I wasn't changing what was causing my cancer, and it was my job to figure it out and change it if I wanted to survive it. I'm also not saying that those who don't find what's causing their cancer won't overcome it. People do. Maybe they never knew what caused their cancer, but whatever the cause was got resolved between the time they were diagnosed, and the time they were cured. It's even possible that the harsh effects of traditional treatments helped them. Was it the treatments that cured them, or was it a coincidence and they would have been cured anyway? Was it psychosomatics? If you ask them, most will swear it was the treatments that saved them.

135

The power of belief can take us anywhere.

I never believed in the chemo I was given. I don't think it ever could have helped me beyond the first treatments. Others who have the same belief as me, probably should not be using it as a treatment option, either. It's a dreadfully hard decision to make. Especially when nearly everyone is on the chemo bandwagon and support for those stepping outside the standards of care is non-existent. All I can say is we have to make our own choices and be brave in those decisions. It doesn't belong to anyone else. Then we should seek support for that decision, and run with it. If we change our minds later on, then that's even better. We just need to take our time, and not make the decisions under other people's pressures. Make well researched, educated decisions, and have confidence in those decisions. Just don't feel trapped in one frame of mind. I believe that if one treatment isn't working after a few months, it may be time to switch it to something else.

In the beginning, my doctors and family wanted me to do the standard treatments, and I was never even asked whether I wanted to do something else. It was just naturally assumed I would go along with the standards of care because there was nothing else they could offer me. I dragged my feet about it, but I chose to do them entirely out of fear and desperation. My hope in doing them was that my suffering would be eliminated quickly, which didn't even happen.

I didn't allow any outside factors to influence my decision the second time around. By then, I had done the research, and I had seen the effects chemo was having on the people I knew and on myself, as well. I was dead certain chemo would be the end of me. As a result of going with my instinct, my body was able to keep beating the cancer back.

I would never tell a cancer patient NOT to do chemo or radiation if that is what they wanted to do. If they truly believe the treatments can cure their cancer, it just might! If they're leery about it at all, maybe another choice would be better, or do like I did and give it a single go. Knowledge is power, so I can only suggest to continually do research! I will list as much helpful information as I can in the appendix of this book.

My chemo treatments hadn't worked, so my oncologist recommended we try a different type of chemo. He had my personal cancer cells tested against all the different types of chemo and he said my cancer responded positively to every chemo available. The only question I had for him after hearing that was why didn't the first chemo kill all the cancer then? His response both amazed, and terrified me. He said sometimes the cancer cells get used to the chemo (immune to it), and then it no longer kills them. Then they would have to switch to another chemo. Under that theory, logically, it would be fair for me to assume that the cancer would never fully be killed. It would just keep mutating and strengthening until nothing on Earth could stop it. In the meantime, my quality of life would plummet and I would die a slow, miserable death as either all my organs started failing from the toxic chemicals my body was constantly flooded with, or the cancer over-ran my body. No. No, no, no, no, no.

I began to realize that chemo most likely worked, but the dosage needed to destroy every cancer cell floating around would destroy the patient, as well. As it was, the every-other-week doses patients were given was already enough to kill them. I attribute it to dropping a nuclear bomb on a civil war. Both sides lose.

Was it a big risk to opt out of chemo treatments after getting a metastatic diagnosis? It was a much bigger risk for me to do chemo treatments, as far as I was concerned. But I also understood why someone else would believe otherwise. When a medical professional tells you this is what we have, and there is nothing else, you tend to believe them. Why wouldn't you?

When I was first diagnosed, all I wanted was the cancer out of me. Each subsequent recurrence was the same...just cut it out of me!

The chemo and radiation shrank my tumor and saved my rectum the first time around. It was more beneficial under those circumstances to do the treatments. However, if I had known then, what I know now, I might not have done the six months of adjuvant chemo I got after my first surgery. Hindsight is 20/20. I would not have known how ineffective the chemo was for me for certain, if I hadn't done the adjuvant chemo. All in all, it was a good choice I never regretted.

The only thing I can say to someone newly diagnosed is do the research and don't make any hasty decisions, at all. Cancer can be time sensitive, of course, but as I've said before, I believe it's never too late to find your personal cure, and many things will probably be tried before it's figured out. There is time.

Finding the purpose to my cancer was an important step in healing and helped strengthen my belief that I could heal on my own terms.

I always believed that everything happens for a

purpose. As cliché as it sounds, I saw correlations in my life events that were too specific to be random. Such as people I'd meet, who for some reason, taught me something I really needed to know right when I needed to learn it. Meeting David six months before I got really sick is the perfect example of such an event. I often wondered what I would have done, or how I would've survived if he hadn't entered my life at that time. I also saw the benefit I had in his life. David is an avid vegetarian and a much more conscientious person than before I met him. We came into each-other's lives, gave each other what the other one needed, then graciously stepped aside. I just love how life is set up that way. There are patterns like puzzle pieces that naturally fall into place in order for us to succeed. We just have to pay attention and follow the signs. If we stray off-course, something always seems to happen to guide us back onto the right course. At least that's how it's always been for me. Aside from the obvious, there seems to be something very intentional in the way things naturally work.

Cancer, to me, isn't any different than any other life teacher. It has purpose, and in my life, the purpose was in many lessons. I was running around in my life as a total stress case. Every time something went wrong, I'd react very negatively to it and that kept me in a constant state of unhappiness and frustration. My marriage failing put me into a fit of personal chaos. The cancer came and forced me to change my life. Now I'm a much better person for it. It put me in the position to gain control of my spiraling unhappy life, and put me on course with how I really wanted my life to go. What better purpose is there than that? Well, for me, I can tell you one other great situation that adds to the positive purpose of my cancer; no one else in my family should ever get this disease if they stay on top of their colonoscopies. Colorectal cancer is one of the most preventable cancers known. A plucked polyp during a colonoscopy can mean the difference between cancer, and no cancer; between life, and possible premature death.

I don't think cancer is a lesson anyone is raising their hands and volunteering to learn, but since we have it, we might as well open the door, and peer in to see what its offering.

Remember the power play on the word cancer that I talked about earlier. We CAN beat cancer by changing our Conditioned Emotional Responses to it.

CAN C.E.R. does not control me. I control it.

CAN C.E.R. is not a death sentence. It's a wake-up call.

CAN C.E.R. is an opportunity to change my life for the better.

CAN C.E.R. is my body's way of telling me I'm not living up to my potential.

CAN C.E.R. Will not destroy my life, it is a personal challenge to improve my life and learn how to take responsibility for my own health and happiness.

I began looking at my cancer journey as an adventure very early on. It's never too late to look at it in that way, because that's exactly what it is. It's an adventure not only into experiencing things most other people do not, but an adventure into learning about myself and an opportunity to improve myself. It's a means to enrich my own life in unimaginable ways. This is my opportunity to see how strong and resilient my body and spirit really is. That is another gift not everyone in life is given.

Cancer makes us VERY aware of our bodies and its systems. How many people know the function of the liver, let alone which side of the body it's on?
People with liver cancer or mets to the liver know these things.

Knowing our bodies is a good step in learning how to communicate with our bodies. Communication between mind and body is a good idea for keeping the body healthy and functional and for figuring out what is going on inside our bodies that we might not know otherwise.

I'm lucky that I have a very vocal body and my mind/body connection is
naturally very strong. I think a lot of us in today's day and age have lost touch of that connection with our busy lives, unhealthy eating habits, and poor sleeping patterns.
Getting that connection back will greatly help in healing.

Just before my diagnosis, I developed the oddest craving for pickles and engine exhaust. For weeks I'd eat jar upon jar of pickles. I was eating on average, four jars a week of a food I'd never really cared for in the past.

As far as the engine exhaust goes, well that was just the strangest thing of all! I'd sneak out of the house late at night to stick my nose under the hood of one of the cars to get a good, deep whiff of it. I would have dreams about the smell and wake up craving it. I hid a bottle of engine oil in the kitchen cupboard that I'd have to sniff dozens of times throughout the day.

Oddly enough, after my first blood transfusion, both cravings almost instantly ended. I don't know to this day why being anemic caused the bizarre cravings, but the point is that my body was screaming for something it

141

desperately needed, and that was how it communicated it.

There are easier ways to figure out what our bodies need without it having to scream out in desperation.

Finding quiet moments in our lives where we can relax and concentrate on ourselves can build that bridge to a mind/body connection. Meditating on a question we have for our body will yield results, too. Once we can put ourselves into a meditative state where all outside interference is blocked out and only silence remains, we can ask our body a question, and an answer will come from within.

Through my experimentation with meditation and lucid dreaming, both have worked accurately for a number of issues. Even solving math questions while I was in college were done successfully during lucid dreaming. There are plenty of books on how to do meditation, but without getting too demonstrative with it, I can say that different methods work for different people. I started doing it while lying in bed before going to sleep. I'd light a bunch of candles and burn my favorite incense, and then I'd lay there quietly concentrating on silencing my mind. It takes a lot of practice to quiet the mind, and I fell asleep a couple of times during my first few attempts, but once it's accomplished for even a few seconds, the most calming peace overcomes the mind. Putting a CD on with repetitive drum beats can help with the relaxation, and concentration, too.

Another way I practice calming the mind is I close my eyes and count as high as I can without another thought entering my mind. As soon as some thought other than the numbers comes into my mind, I start over. I kept practicing until I could reach a higher number. This exercise really helped with opening up new perceptions of thought. Once I was able to quiet my mind, I was able to commune with my body and found de-stressing easier. It's a challenge to not get frustrated when the mind refuses to find quiet for very long. The mind can only be completely quiet for fractions of a second at a time. The point in attempting to quiet the mind is to train the mind to focus on one thing at a time while shutting out the distractions that break concentration and communication. The more practice in quieting the mind, the better control there will be on outside influences while communicating with the body.

While in a relaxed, open-minded state, ask the body a question over and over again, thinking of nothing else. If there is no interference, the answer will come.

Yoga is another way to get in closer touch with the body. Though yoga can be challenging for people whose body have been altered through surgeries and long down periods, there is chair yoga and even phone yoga classes particular for people with cancer.

I had developed a mild atrophy of the muscles in my upper legs and buttocks that bothers me to this day. Any stretching of the muscles in those particular areas causes a lot of pain, but I still attempt to stretch the area two or three times per day.

With yoga, and any exercise, be cautious of any limitations, and slowly work through them, if any. I took some chair yoga at the cancer center during my treatments that was very helpful.

Chi Gong (Qi Gong), or Tai Chi, are two beautiful forms of movement that can really help with a mind/body connection, and the former is particularly great for people with cancer. Ask your TCM (traditional Chinese) doctor about where these classes are held and check senior centers in your area. You don't have to be a senior to take classes there.

The added bonus to these types of exercises are, the great stress relieving benefits they have. In fact, any type of exercise is going to help relieve stress, if not overdone. I found that whenever I over did myself with exercise, it would cause set-backs to my routine, sometimes very long set-backs. It was hard for me to judge exactly when I was pushing too hard usually until it was too late. I learned my limitations by going into any new type of exercise gradually, whether I felt like I could do more, or not. A five minute walk one day, a ten minute walk the next, then a day off to test recovery time.

Cancer certainly has purpose for all of us, no matter what it is. Whether we're the ones who have it, or the ones who know someone who has it, it brings us closer as communities rally for support, and loved ones gather together to help each other out. Cancer forces us to feel our compassion and mercy, and therefore enables us to better relate to each other on a higher level of consciousness. It can save the lives of others who've been affected by our journey by bringing awareness and education to the subject. It can open and/or alter our perceptions about life and direct us to a different path of existence we didn't even know was possible.

13.
THE KEY TO THE REPAIR

Belief is $4/10^{th}$ of the law, and nutrition is $2/10^{th}$ of the law in my formula for beating cancer. The remaining $4/10$'s of the law has proved overall, to be the most important aspect for me in my healing.

The key to my cure quite simply is happiness.

I don't mean the fleeting happiness that comes as a result of a special event on a sunny day that can be taken away when the rain comes and spoils it. I'm talking about the happiness that comes from pure inner contentment.

With stress being my trigger, I couldn't achieve contentment until I had peace in my living situation and elimination of all my overwhelming stress.

I was happy when I lived with my grandmother; especially during the last year while I was with Chris, but I still had a high degree of stress that was too intense to give me contentment. As soon as that last bit of stress was eliminated (when I moved out of my grandmother's house, and finally had total freedom of body and mind), was I able to fall into the ultimate contentment and happiness phase.

Discovering my joy and creating my own happiness was, and continues to be, the most adventuresome and exciting part of healing and living that I've ever experienced. I have a natural euphoria every day and an insatiable desire to taste life like never before. That's the point, after all!

So how does one go about finding happiness?

Well, first of all, understanding what happiness through contentment is is the way I achieved it. I realized it wasn't something that can really be found, like something that was lost, or even like something that can be acquired by looking outside of myself. It's a state of mind and it started with the realization that I was the one in control of my emotions and that I was the one with the choice to create that state of mind by simply caring for myself and my needs.

I decided that my life was great just as it was, and it would only get better from there. By deciding there was only reason for joy and happiness to exist in my life, I began the journey to gaining it. If I look at all the negatives as having positive outcomes, I would feel satisfaction out of as many events as possible, even the not so great ones. While living with my grandmother, I kept this tidbit in my mind, constantly; that someday soon, my life would change for the better, even though I didn't know at the time how to change it, just having that goal in my mind led me to the change.

I'm not saying I became Pollyanna or one of those people who have a false sense of optimism about every aspect of life. Everyone has less than great days from time to time, and everyone feels blue here and again. It's perfectly natural to have those emotions and to express them appropriately. Feel them, for sure, then when that time passes, come up with a game plan and move on. Every problem has a solution and I always kept in mind that seemingly negative events lead to something positive, even if it's a chain of negative events. I don't allow ANYTHING to steal my joy. I embrace every moment, good or bad, and remind myself that only good can come from both types of events. If there is something that is robbing me of my happiness, I make a new plan. Remind myself over and over again that I deserve to be happy. Train my mind to accept it. Even when I'm in a bad mood, or a sad mood, which happens sometimes, I do something I know will make me feel better (like listen to a particular song, or watch a special movie), or get a hold of someone I trust, and tell them how I'm feeling. I remind myself how wonderful the air tastes, or the day looks. I do whatever it takes, and if none of that helps, then I know I need to allow myself to experience the grief longer, then move on from it when I'm ready. In moments where I get angry with myself and tell myself that I'm not deserving of happiness, I remind myself that this is just a moment in a sea of moments, and it too, will pass.

It isn't always easy to remember these steps, and I consciously tell myself that it's okay to feel the way I'm feeling when I feel bad, but I remind myself that inside I'm happy, and even though I'm not feeling happy at that particular moment, I know I will feel happiness again soon. I mentally list the reasons why I'm happy, and what I have to be grateful for. I take deep breaths where I can feel the air hit the base of my lungs, and I'm thankful that I still have 1.5 lungs. I do so love the taste of air! I go outside and either let the sun beat down on my face for a few seconds, or let the rain or cold air beat down on me. I experience whatever nature is doing on the day I'm finding difficulty, and find solace in the ability to feel it. I hug my animals and tell them I love them, and sometimes cry while I'm cuddling them tight because I love them so much. Particularly my pugs, Rainbow and Oliver, bring me such great joy. I have Rainbow trained and registered as my emotional support animal, and she is a great addition to my contentment. The people I care about make me tremendously happy, too, most of the time! But it isn't really these outside influences that make me happy so much as it's my ability to feel these things.

I make every adjustment I can to continually add happiness to ALL aspects of my life and eliminate the factors that threaten it.

I know a lot of people are used to the grind and stress of their jobs and go about their day mundanely, miserably, difficultly, or all the above. Days turn into weeks, and the weekend is the highlight of their lives. The thought of another Monday coming depresses them immensely.

If a person feels this way about their job, either a change of job is in order, or their emotional response to their job must change. The job or working environment is where most people spend the majority of their lives. How can we possibly be happy if we hate, or are in any way uncomfortable with where we spend the majority of our waking hours?

Whether someone decides to change their job, or change the way they view their job, either choice can be stressful. It doesn't have to be, though. Just remember the CAN C.E.R. Motto. We can change our emotional responses. This applies to every aspect of our lives, not just the disease. If we decide to stay at our unhappy job, we must ask ourselves why we're unhappy with it, and what changes could be made to make it more tolerable. If it's outside influences making us unhappy, such as

148

conflict with a co-worker or boss, what is it that makes them intolerable? How can we change our responses to their behavior or interactions? We make a conscious decision to create a happy environment for ourselves, regardless of those around us. We have a plan about how we're going to react to the situation, and have the confidence to play it out. By making that one, simple, decision, a feeling of relief starts to come over us. I am in charge of how I feel, and how I allow others to make me feel. I try to remember to always stay calm during confrontations. The tone of my own voice can seriously set the tone for the entire confrontation. If my voice is soft and controlled, the angry person's voice will eventually calm down, too. I've used this technique with VERY agro people who go into fits of rage, and it's worked. The only plan I had was that when she confronted me, I wasn't going to react. Her rage was her own, and had nothing whatsoever to do with me. Approaching it in that way separated my emotions from hers, and kept my blood pressure and heart-rate down to normal levels. This was one of many skills I learned from Chris. After the confrontation, I didn't need any calm down time and I felt so good about myself for not allowing myself to be affected by someone else's emotions. That strengthened my confidence and made me feel more in control of my environment.

Stress, like I've mentioned before, and will say a thousand times if
necessary is NOT the way to happiness. It's not even a true necessity in our lives. The fight or flight response in us is over used to the point of breeding cancer cells and promoting all kinds of other illnesses. There is an amazing

book written called Buddha's Brain that explains this wonderful phenomenon, and other interesting facts about our intricate brains (see appendix). The fight or flight response in humans is a primitive adaptation we needed back in the caveman days, but don't need now. When we were in serious danger, or facing a life-threatening situation, an adrenaline surge would kick in, flooding our systems with stress hormones so we could react in the appropriate manner: Either kick some serious trash, or RUN like the devil's on our heels.

Several tens of thousands of years later, we no longer have any natural predators, and no longer really need the fight or flight response. However, it is still in us, and we still use it. Unfortunately, we use it all the time, and primarily in situations where it is completely unnecessary. Such as having an argument with a loved one, or worrying about a confrontation at work. For many of us, we allow these little situations to trigger the fight or flight response in us. We worry about the event, and perseverate about it, sometimes to the point of losing sleep. Using this response keeps our bloodstreams flooded with stress hormones and in a revved up, uncomfortable state where our immune systems are continually being kept busy fighting those unnecessary battles. While that's going on, serious illnesses and diseases that are festering on the sidelines go unchecked and are allowed to gain control of the body. Changing our responses from fight or flight, to calm, cool, and collected, will greatly reduce the stress hormones in the body, and thus free up our immune systems to work successfully as the disease sentinels they're designed to be.

Again, this may take some practice, but keeping in

mind that our life is on the line, and that responding reactively to any situation is not worth our life, can be a great motivator in keeping our cool. It has sure worked well for me. I'm sometimes calmer than I probably should be in some situations.

I'm not suggesting that we should be complacent when someone is screaming in our face, or on the verbal attack. When things get that heated, respond calmly, or don't respond at all. Leave the situation without a reaction, especially if the conflict seems serious enough to get violent. Be self-assertive without aggression, and deal with the situation in an alternative way.

Being self-assertive is a great way to feel really good about ourselves, too.

I was a type beta-personality, which basically means I avoided confrontations and was generally the type of person who would rather let things slide, than get into a big fight over them. I was the type of person who would not want to make anyone displeased, or feel like I was being rude to them. Not the self-assertive type of personality, at all. I think this is the personality type that is prone to getting cancer. I've witnessed many times a different personality type in which the person is overly self-assertive, and aggressive in what they want. The people I've seen with this alpha-personality type seem to have more health issues with their hearts.

I don't want to be either of those personality types, but I do want to be able to stick up for myself when I'm being wronged and to not feel like I always have to be the one getting taken advantage of. I've learned how to properly do that without causing stress on myself, and instead, make each of those moments, moments of empowerment.

151

In doing this, I've found that it not only makes me feel wonderful about myself, but it starts a chain of positive Karma in my life.

It should be an act that doesn't require much thought, but I have always struggled with being self-assertive.

My grandmother's caregivers were always running all over me because they instinctively knew this. They would often times rearrange items in the house, or take the liberty of organizing a system in the kitchen that worked for them, regardless of the fact that other people lived there. I can't say how much time I wasted searching for something as simple as a measuring cup, but it was too much, that's for sure!

The best examples of being self-assertive that pertains to self-advocacy, is at doctor's offices.

I remember when I was first having the tailbone issues and the doctors and nurses kept putting me off and making their own assumptions of the situation when I knew something more serious was going on. It took putting my foot down and insisting on seeing a specialist that finally got me the right diagnosis. I wasn't rude about it, I simply asked for the referral, and told my oncologist that I wasn't satisfied with the results I was getting so far.

I'm no longer meek about asking for what I want and need. If they tell me no, I don't necessarily stop there, either. I never get aggressive about it. I never raise my voice; in fact, I have no emotional attachment to the outcome at all, if I can help it. If something really important goes awry, I simply handle it as it has to be handled, like when the insurance switched on me a week before my lung surgery.

There's no reason to stress out about any situation

unless the flight or fight response is a warranted situation. Like a car accident or an unexpected attack. I learned this when my relationship with Chris ended in the manner I described in another chapter. It was a very unexpected attack that caught me completely off-guard. It was over the phone, almost identical to the scenario that occurred with my ex-husband nearly a decade earlier. Just like the time before, I almost instantly had a nervous breakdown that was very similar to the first one. I think it was exemplified simply because it was such a déjà vu moment.

At any rate, the response my body had to the shock was nearly identical to the first time it happened. There were only two differences. Instead of the paralysis in my legs preventing me from walking for fifteen minutes, I lost the feeling in my left leg for four months and it never fully recovered. The other difference was the cancer was found a few months later rather than two years later.

Though the experience was painful and stressful, it wasn't as bad as the first time it had happened. I was in shock, for sure, but it was mostly shock that history had repeated itself in such an exacting manner.

The one thing I'd always sensed about Chris throughout our time together was that he was not an honest or trustworthy person. He had accomplished a lot in his life and had experienced some horrendous things along the way; the types of things that either made someone a good person, or ruined any chance of that ever happening. No matter how many sweet words and promises he fed me, I could never bring myself to fully trust him. There were just too many red-flags and strange occurrences that kept me forever on my guard. Still, I gave him the benefit of the doubt, hoping my instincts were wrong. Sadly, everything I'd feared about him ended up revealing itself all in a single moment.

The experience took a toll on me that took a while to recover from, but during the healing process, I never lost my inner contentment or overall happiness with my life. One of the things Chris always demanded of me (something that also kept me leery of him), was that he wanted me to rely on him for my happiness. I thought it was a strange thing to request; especially since he requested it often, and I always had the same response to it. I told him he could only add to my happiness. If I didn't have inner happiness, it wouldn't be real.

Knowing who Chris is now, I often wonder if he was so desperate for my happiness simply so he could rob me of it. I know it sounds paranoid, but the manner in which he ended our relationship (the same way my marriage ended), and the fact that he knew the event caused my original cancer, makes it all look very purposeful. Another clue that his actions were intentional is that he's continued, just up until this past July, to contact me, always inquiring about my health. I have never had the slightest urge to respond. Not in anger, and not in peace. I don't regret getting involved with him and I harbor no bitterness. I learned a lot from the experience and it's made me a better, and much more enlightened, person. He did add to my happiness for a short time, but when he left, my happiness didn't go with him. Not by a long shot.

Sorry Chris, if you want to know that I survived you, you have to buy the book. *smiley face*

All kidding aside, I have no room in my life for those who would purposely or otherwise try to rob me of my happiness. They couldn't anyway because happiness isn't

154

something that can be given or taken away by someone else. Anyone who thinks that's possible hasn't found their inner happiness yet. That's okay. It can be found with just a little self-analysis and a lot of blatant, personal truths. I'll get to that in a moment.

I will mention here that sometimes there are people in our lives who seem to bring a dark cloud with them everywhere they go. They feel like a dark energy of grief that thickens the air, surrounding us with a negative vibe. All I can say is get away from these people no matter who they are. When dealing with a life-threatening illness, it's very important for us to have good energy around us, and people who make us laugh and celebrate. There is no room for the other type of people. I don't feel bad cutting these people from my life. In fact, I feel like a weight has been lifted. Whenever I find myself trapped with a dark cloud person, I mentally surround myself in a protective bubble that emotionally separates me from them that they cannot penetrate.

Another component for happiness through contentment that I'm a strong proponent of is subsistent living. What I mean by that is everyone should be able to make their living doing what they love based on their skills and talents. This may be a very utopian and idealistic way of thinking, but look at it this way; people ARE doing it, and if any one person in this world can do it, we ALL can! The only thing different between the people who make their living doing what they love, and those who don't, is the ones who are, have the confidence, determination and motivation to do it. That's it. They want it, they believe they can do it without any doubt, and they go for it. To me, achieving high success is simply the inability to

155

understand failure. In other words, do, and do, and do, again. As Yoda says, "...there is no try." It may not happen all at once, but it can't fail if you keep trying. Just try new ways of accomplishing it. Okay, so not everyone can be a professional basketball player no matter how badly they want it, but surely there's something else that person is passionate about. If not, more self-analysis and trial and error is in order. Struggling to achieve a goal that is completely out of reach isn't going to make us happy. I believe everyone has multiple things they're good at that brings them joy, so settling on just one of those things won't always work.

My favorite quote regarding this way of thinking is from Walt Disney. To paraphrase what he said; "If you can dream it, you can achieve it." Just look at the empire that one man created, all from a single dream and the 'knowledge' he could do it.

We are all capable of realizing our dreams. All it takes is confidence, determination and motivation. Some people have this naturally, and others of us have to consciously develop it. The good news is we CAN all do it. It's another superpower we all have and can tap into.

Another way to happiness through contentment, is by expressing our creativity in any way that brings us joy and doing it every chance we get. No matter what it is, if it gives us joy (and it's not hurting anyone), it's a great thing! Fulfilling our passions on a daily basis is extremely healthy. Have more than one? Do them all! The more the merrier!

I had a ton of activities I loved to do, or desired to someday do, but most of them felt out of reach for me for a very long time either because of my weight, or because

156

of illness, or finances, or time, or I thought I wasn't good enough, or whatever excuse worked at the time. Going to Disneyland was one of my favorite things to do, but the excuse I was using for not going, was my health, and the expense.

The first time I went back after my initial surgery I had earned a free pass doing simple volunteer work for a non-profit organization and spent the day at the park being pushed around in a wheelchair by my best friend. It was a fun day, but I wasn't able to fully enjoy it. I feared going on the roller coasters because of the tailbone issue, and I worried the whole day that Aaron was ruining his hands pushing the wheelchair around. It was one of the big eye opening motivators of my life. I decided that day that I wasn't going to spend my life in a wheelchair. I had to be whole again so I could walk on my own, and go on the roller coasters again. I also decided I would continue to find ways to afford it, whether I had to save every penny for a time, or win a ticket like I had before. It became a passionate goal, and I started taking small walks every night. I started off slowly, first just walking continually around the house, then to the top of the street, then around the block. Eventually I was able to join the gym and swim regularly. I also financed a Disneyland season pass.

After a few months, and one more trip to Disneyland needing a wheelchair, I never needed one again. My tailbone is still problematic and causes me a lot of agony at times, but I'm able to go to water parks and do roller coasters without the aid of a wheelchair, and I even got to a point where I could do Zumba classes at the gym. The neuropathy in my legs has prevented me from being able to do the classes anymore, but at least I can still walk.

I know my capabilities well, but not always my limits. I still get to the point where I'm incapacitated if I do too much, but I'm always working to overcome my physical challenges. I don't let it depress me when I can't do something, and if I do get a little down, I take every effort in turning that around. Life is just too precious to squander it on self-pity for too long. I give myself a day to wallow, and then I snap out of it. I desire happiness, so I have it.

Feeling useful added to my contentment, too. Not just useful, but needed. My grandmother needed me and at times it was very rewarding being able to take care of her. Unfortunately, there were far too many other influences surrounding that situation, like being taken advantage of by family members, to make it a healthy type of usefulness for me. When I started fostering homeless pug dogs through Pug Rescue of San Diego County, I really began feeling the healthy type of usefulness. Being a devoted animal lover and having a super soft spot for pugs in particular, nothing felt better than giving them a loving place to be while I got to choose the best possible home for them.

Volunteering occasionally or anything that gives the feeling of making a difference in the community or in the world, can be so very fulfilling. It nurtures confidence, causes euphoria, and gives purpose.

Sometimes we have to learn what our limitations are and stay within those limitations to keep the stress down and the happiness flowing. Taking on too much can have the complete opposite effect, such as it did with me with my grandmother.

In the cancer circle I'm a part of, I see this with so

158

many other people. Particularly with women, but it pertains to men in the same situation as well.

I see them dealing with their cancer while expending themselves to the point of exhaustion for their family. I see this as a conundrum for them; torn between neglecting their family's needs, and doing what they need to do for themselves in order to heal.

The women I've talked to about this express a deep desire to get off the chemo because they're sick all the time, and find it difficult to live productive family lives. They think that ending chemo treatments is the same as giving up and letting the cancer win.

First of all, switching gears is NOT giving up. Switching gears is exactly what's needed in a case like this, whether it's giving up chemo, or just by eliminating the stress.

Family members and loved ones can put a lot of pressure on us inadvertently and it's our responsibility as the only people who know what we need, to tell them our limitations and learn to say no sometimes. Being assertive and standing up for ourselves doesn't mean we're being selfish. It doesn't mean we're not being nice, and no one will like us for it. It means we want to live.

One of my colorectal cancer friends who was diagnosed a stage IV at the age of 43, had four kids between 8-18 years old. We would have lengthy conversations about this very subject. I was constantly trying to get her to slow down and rest. She was always so exhausted and always had schedules to follow for one kid or the other. There were always soccer games, ballet lessons, and band practice to drive them to. She had the responsibility of cooking all the meals and keeping up the household. She was too tired to make the meals they wanted as well as the healthy food she wanted to eat, so it was her needs that got sidelined time and time again. She always talked about wanting to start juicing, or wanting to begin one healthy diet or another, but her kids wouldn't eat that kind of food. It was either what they wanted, or nothing. She was too worn out and sick to do both. Of course a good Mother and wife would always believe it was her duty to choose her family over herself. I can understand this mentality, completely. However, it's an illogical and counterproductive choice when we're sick. Our family will struggle temporarily without us while we take the time to heal ourselves, but they will struggle for the rest of their lives if we die. The person who's going to take care of our family when we die, needs to be the person stepping up to the plate while we heal. Who is that person? Is it our spouse, our own parent/s, our in-laws, our kids, our neighbors, themselves? We need to be assertive, ask these people for help now! Our kids will have a lot of fast growing up to do, but at least they'll grow up with us still here and they won't have to deal with growing up too fast because their parent died.

My friend's family is struggling to figure out exactly how they're going to exist now because she didn't heal from her cancer. She passed away at the young age of 45.

This story illustrates how a lot of people are having to deal with their illness. My friend is not the only person who has told me a similar story. I truly believe that my friend's life would have been prolonged or spared if she had been able to take care of herself as she needed to.

By using my friend's story as an example, maybe I can reach others in this same situation and make them realize that putting themselves first while they heal from their disease is not abandoning their family. It's quite the opposite. By taking care of themselves now, they will be around for many years to come. That is what their family really needs; for them to be there for many more years to come. For myself, I knew while I was in the situation with my grandmother that it wasn't a place conducive to my health. I felt trapped by obligation with very few options. If my aunt hadn't kicked me out, I don't know how many recurrences it would've taken before I left, or if the cancer would have just overcome me altogether. If a situation is too stressful; work, living situation, family...it must be changed. It must! We must sit down with our loved ones, and lay it out. I didn't do that, but was very fortunate that events turned the way they did and I was forcibly removed from the situation. It was exactly what I needed and I know now that that one single event is most likely what saved my life.

Here is another example of possibly doing too much.

My oncologist had asked me to be a patient advocate for the cancer center and I definitely wanted to do it. I wasn't going to do it until I was in a healthy place in my life and health, first. When I was certain that I could be around people in my situation without it stressing me out with grief, and risk my own demise, then I would do it.

I knew better than to get involved in cancer causes while I was trying to heal. Being reminded constantly that people were dying of this and being put into a state of grief all the time, was NOT an emotionally healthy place for me to be. I knew once I was in a healthy emotional and physical place, I would write this book, and hopefully help others in my situation. If cancer is all around us while we're trying to heal, it's hard for us to focus on what's outside of cancer, which is health, longevity, and contentment; some of the very important items we need in order to heal. It's not healthy to hear people constantly complaining about how horrible cancer is, and that they wished it didn't exist. It DOES exist, and those who are always pointing out how horrible it is aren't helping anything for anybody.

I've been guilty of spreading less than joyous comments about cancer myself, in the past, so I can't blame anyone else for doing it. Those of us who want in a different place, though, should go to a different place.

While needing to heal, it's important to let anyone and everyone help out with family responsibilities. The grandparents can help in many cases, or the spouse can take on more responsibility. Find help if there is no one else around. Moving closer to those who will help you can be an option. Communicate to those who are around and let them know what they can do to help in order for you to recover your health. Most people are eager and anxious to help out. Sometimes it's the family members who feel the most helpless when a loved one gets cancer. Remember that life will continue without us when we die, so let it continue without us while we heal, instead. Sit down with a caregiver and discuss options. The family can join in eating healthy meals, it won't kill them, but eating otherwise might kill us. Have neighbors, or the kid's friend's parents take the kids to school. Have the confidence to ask for help, and most importantly, NEVER feel guilty about it. We'll have plenty of time to make it up to those who helped us after we've healed, particularly by doing the same for someone else in need.

If there is any way we can convalesce while healing, we must by all means do it. Take part in activities that are stress relieving, not stress inducing. This might seem difficult to do at first, but just like everything else, it all starts with a decision, then a plan, then executing the plan over and over again. Our lives get turned upside down with a cancer diagnosis, so while it's already upside down, make whatever necessary changes needed to get into a healing position when things go right side up again.

The local cancer center or treatment facility probably offers services such as social workers and psychologists, and there are other resources that could help, like cancercare.com, and the American Cancer Society. Being our own assertive advocates is a sure fire step to health and happiness and it also aids in reducing stress.

If we make friends with other people who are in a similar situation as us, by all means we should spend time with them. It's so nice to have people around us who understand what we're going through! We just shouldn't spend our time together focusing on the cancer. Instead we should participate in activities that distract from the challenges of the illness and bring good times and memories we can look back on in our times of distress. Each one of those moments is a healing, stress-free, moment.

Making lists of goals will help with organization, and can seriously reduce stress. Lists are especially important for anyone doing any kind of hard core cancer treatments. I quickly developed chemo brain and found it difficult to concentrate on anything for very long. My memory was especially affected. I highly recommend lists for everyone, though.

Lists not only helped with my forgetfulness, but knowing I didn't have to store so much information in my already saturated brain, let me actually relax into my day.

A general list could be similar to this;

1. As soon as I wake up, I look out the window, and thank the Universe

for another day of life (expressing gratitude reminds us that we're thankful to be

alive).

2. Do five chair squats, and five arm lifts as soon as I rise from bed.

3. Take morning vitamins.

4. Make fresh, organic juice.

5. While drinking (and chewing) juice slowly, make a list of today's

planned activities, and/or doctors appointments, phone calls to make,

transportation schedules, etc.

5. Meditation time, bath time, or other "me" time.

6. Bed time, 10 PM .

Lists will improve and become more organized with practice. I learned how to make sub-lists from my general lists, and I also learned to make duplicates of lists to have in more than one place.

Lists not only keep me organized and free up my mind for other things, but they help me stay focused.

The one thing I never say anymore is that I don't have time for the things I need to do to heal. I make the time. In fact, it's the thing I spend the most of my time on. Making lists of how I'm going to take care of myself is something

164

I have notebooks full of.

I make lists of detailed meal plans from the recipes in my myriad of cookbooks or I create my own, like the ones in the back of this book. Creating meal plans can be a great activity that can be done including the whole family. Kids love being active and especially young children love feeling useful. An added bonus is the quality time spent together and that they'll be learning how to take care of themselves when they're grown, and/or how to take care of their beloved parents, when they need down time.

Lists can be general, lists can be detailed, lists can even remind us to practice our calm and our cool. Lists bring a feeling of being productive, even if everything on the list wasn't completed. Just being able to cross one thing off of a list feels great! Maybe the next day, two things will get crossed off. Practice makes better, and better is stress-free!

There's contentment.

Greet the new day with gratitude. I have the perspective of realizing my mortality. This is definitely a blessing to count, and I write them all down, regularly. Seek out what it is that makes others with cancer feel like having it is a gift.

I mentioned the gifts of cancer earlier. Recounting our cancer gifts gives us power over the illness, and makes us feel good about ourselves. I can't illustrate enough how important feeling good about ourselves is when recovering from a life-threatening illness. If the gifts can't be easily seen, search for them. I'm sure they're there, somewhere.

I feel better now with metastatic cancer, than I've ever felt in my life! I have more energy and I have learned how to truly be thankful for my own life. Those feelings didn't happen overnight.

Whatever gifts cancer gives us, it's very personal, but they are there. Discovering the gifts of cancer changed the way I viewed my cancer. I could no longer look at it as "the beast", or "The Dreaded Monster" that I'd forever be fighting. Yes, it was something that I had to beat back, but I couldn't look

at it as something negative. Once I understood the point of it, I understood the good of it.

Seeing so many of my friends and acquaintances die of it no longer angered me or made me hate cancer. It made me sad and it motivated me to do my part to make a change. I believed that I had information that could save lives, and it was my responsibility to get it out there.

Once the fear and anger is gone, we can begin to realize cancer's gifts to us. The anger and fear must go away for healing and survival to take place. When I stopped fearing death, I stopped fearing most other things and my mind and energy was freed to experience life in a different way...such as experiencing contentment, and feeling happiness.

I do anything and everything that will aid and improve the quality of my happiness.

I talked earlier about self-analysis and blatant, personal truths. In order to find inner happiness and contentment, we must take a good, hard, look at ourselves both inside and out.

What do we see when we look at ourselves in the mirror? Do we criticize our appearance harshly, or are we quick to point out the things we don't like about our body, face, hair…? Do we call ourselves 'stupid' and judge ourselves for not being able to remember a task we needed to do, or some other little thing that disappointed us? Do we get bored easily when we're alone? Is that because we can hardly stand being around ourselves? Self-acceptance seems to be one of the hardest things for some of us to achieve, and yet it's such an important aspect in finding inner happiness.

I used to hate my body. Yeah, hate is a strong word, and the way I felt about my body went beyond that. I thought my body sucked for not burning fat the way other people's did, and I hated how misshaped it was; especially after some of the surgeries. There were a dozen things I could point out about my appearance that disgusted me.

It almost makes me laugh now, but it's hardly something that's funny. It's just amazing to me how much I could hate my one-and-only body! My body that defeated cancer how many times? My body that picked itself off the ground when it could barely walk anymore and healed the osteoporosis that was eating through its bones? This body…my body that's been sliced open and stitched up so many times I look like and feel like a ragdoll? This body that without it I could not experience the world or enjoy my pugs, or paint (however badly), or write, or do any of the things I love to do without…?

How could I hate my body?? How can anybody hate their body? The idea is so foreign to me now I almost can't understand it. Yes, my body is misshapen and has a few too many pounds on it. Yes, it's imperfect, but really, it's not imperfect. My body; your body; all of our bodies are an absolute miracle of perfection. Every wrinkle and freckle on my face is a testament to a life lived, and a life experienced. I used to think my nose was too big for my face…maybe it is, but it's MY nose, and I can smell just

167

right with it.

As far as not being able to stand my own company…that has also changed dramatically. I LOVE being alone. I don't know how it all changed, but it started during my separation from my husband. I look forward to being alone so I can write, watch what I want to on TV, paint, or just cuddle with my pugs. I still enjoy being in the company of others, but my alone time is very precious to me.

The simple act of having a clean mouth helps in how I feel about myself, too. Another simple pleasure is painting my nails, and pampering myself. I enjoy cleaning my room, and making it my own special getaway with all the mementos and stuffed animals I've collected and love surrounding myself with. I love having candles and incense burning while I watch a movie. I love exercising now, and that's because of the domino effect of my formula. I find excitement and happiness in the small tasks of my life, which makes the bigger tasks even more enjoyable.

There are so many roads to contentment, it might be infinite. The road I took worked for me, and it will work for others, in their own special mixture. My formula is a guide that can be changed up, developed, improved upon, and combined in any way that will work for the individual.

I once heard happiness described as having something to look forward to. What a wonderful description! Having something to look forward to can be as easy as wondering who that new person in the mirror is going to be when the cancer lesson has ended. Smile, wave, and say hello. Welcome yourself to your new life. If feeling content means quitting that lousy job and living like a bum on the beaches of Tahiti making a living by selling some pieces of palm bark you tied together in the shape of a flower, then heck yeah, go for it!

Contentment is the stable, unwavering happiness that can only be achieved by tapping it from within ourselves. It's being true to ourselves, by realizing our passions, our desires, and by having personal satisfaction with ourselves. It's different for everyone, so only we have the power to give it to ourselves. We accept our situations, even if the acceptance is in changing them, and we embrace who we are as individual pieces of a Universal pie, filled with imperfections, and perfections alike.

Happiness through contentment is the key that opens the door to the cure in my formula.

By eliminating as many factors that cause cancer from our lives as we can, and by identifying our trigger; by eating healthy and taking care of our bodies, and by learning to communicate with them; by knowing we're the ones in control of our own disease, and by having the confidence and bravery to be responsible for our own health; by finding inner happiness through contentment, regardless of outside influences, and by changing emotional responses not only to our disease, but to our surroundings; by utilizing discipline, determination, and motivation to accomplish these above goals, cancer doesn't have a single chance against us! No way!

14.

LOVE & HAPPINESS

Love and happiness…

For some of us, those two words may seem like they don't belong in the same sentence together.

In this society of disposable relationships, I had given up on finding anything genuine in a partner.

In fact, after David and I split up, I knew that getting involved with someone romantically ever again was equivalent to playing Russian roulette with my life. There's nothing like a broken heart to stress someone out to the point of a cancer infestation, right?

It was my belief that because of the serious nature of my illness, no one would be foolish enough to want to get involved with me. Someone even went so far as telling me that once. When I heard that from another person, though, I got angry about it.

Why didn't I deserve love? My future wasn't any more predictable than anybody else's. I had already outlived two people who thought I was going to kick the bucket before they did, and neither one of them had a stage IV cancer diagnosis. One of them was that dear GI doctor who diagnosed me, Dr. Moore.

I may not have been actively looking for love, but I damn well knew I deserved it as much as anyone else did.

I approached dating with an ambivalent attitude, at best. I just wanted to get out there and feel normal again.

Never did I expect, or even really desire, to meet a life partner.

When I met Chris, I was very protective of my feelings for the first year. It was both a fear as much as it was a practicality, though looking back on it I was really scared to death. I was satisfied being single, so I didn't see much of a reason to tempt fate.

It wasn't until I was faced with the lobectomy surgery that I realized I didn't want to live my life in fear of ANYTHING anymore. I was very much in love with Chris, and I made up my mind I was going to nurture that love and enjoy it without the fear of what may, or may not, happen. I couldn't live in fear like that anymore. What else was there really to live for, anyway?

Even though it didn't work out with Chris as I'd hoped, I learned through it that I was still lovable, even with cancer.

Just because we have a serious illness that we're dealing with, doesn't mean we're anything other than lovable. It doesn't mean we're pariah that should be quarantined or isolated so we don't involve others in our lives whom we might hurt if we die. No one is getting out of this life alive, so why live it in fear of death?

Those of us dealing with cancer at any stage who are single and desiring romance in our lives should seriously just go for it! We have the advantage, usually, of knowing who genuine people are when they don't run after they hear the word "cancer", though some just may not care.

When I reached a stage in my life where I was generally happy and feeling good about myself, I attracted

171

someone. I was happy and satisfied, not only personally, but in a comfortable acceptance of my illness. I didn't "need" someone to complete me.

When I first started dating again, I was definitely in the right frame of mind for it. I was emotionally healed, and only had one conundrum; whether or not to tell the people I was dating about the cancer.

I wasn't actively in treatment, and was NED at the time, so it was a burning question I had as to when was the right time, if any, to tell prospective datees about the cancer?

The way I thought about it was that I wasn't looking to get serious with anyone
so it wasn't any of their business. On the other hand, what if I really did meet someone I wanted to be with for the long term? I thought I'd be in quite a spot for not being up front with them about it in the beginning.

The way I feel about it now is that being up front is always the right choice.

Be as open as possible about the cancer, whether it's active, or not, and do it without fear. If they leave right away, they most likely wouldn't have stayed anyway.

Sure, cancer is a very scary thing, but just because we have it, doesn't mean we're going to die from it, no matter what stage it's in.

I got to where I was constantly saying to potential dates that people DO survive cancer!

When I stopped saying that, when I stopped making excuses for why I was dating, that's when I was truly in the zone to attract someone.

Love of any and all kinds, is the fast track way to happiness, contentment, joy, and health! It's all encompassing, and it leads us to alternate perceptions of events, people, and of life in general. I'm talking about all kinds of love, not just love of a partner, or spouse. The love I have for my animals is satisfying, the love for my family, of my own self and of life is satisfying...all of it adds tremendously to my happiness. No, it's more than that. Love IS my happiness.

Touching and being touched is vital not only to our physical health, but critical to our emotional health and happiness. Touch therapy is offered at some spas, and massage therapy, at many cancer centers. I would use these services if I absolutely had to, but I prefer the touch of my loved ones. I highly recommend those of us who are sick, to seek out a dog to bond with, and either train, or have him/her trained to be an emotional support animal. It isn't difficult. I trained Rainbow while I was doing the first rounds of chemo and she's accompanied me to almost all of my doctor appointments, radiation treatments, and even some of my chemo infusions, since she was seven weeks old. The simple act of rubbing her head when I'm stressed calms me immeasurably.

Having love in my heart also releases me from many burdens such as judging others. It is fun practice to look at someone passing by on the street and have absolutely no opinion about them, one way or the other. When we can see people for just what they are...people, we open ourselves up to an entirely new state of perception, and can feel appreciation for our fellow human beings, no matter who they are. It also helps to eliminate another oppressive emotion which is jealousy.

Jealousy, or "The Green-eyed Monster", is exactly what the nick-name implies; a monster. As a perfectly natural emotion, it's one that can quickly turn into something wholly unnatural if it's nurtured and allowed to fester.

In love, and in life, a little jealousy can be motivating and healthy. It's when we dislike others because we're jealous of them, or when we start wishing we were someone we weren't, or worse of all, when we feel we don't deserve what we have, and we're jealous that someone else is going to rob us of it, is when jealousy becomes poisonous and soul oppressing. If we're in a place in our life where we feel we have to covet what someone else has, it's definitely time for a life altering change. Don't be scared, let jealousy and envy go. I am not perfect, but I love the person I am. If I dishonor the good person I am by wishing I was someone I'm not, I'll just be sad and miserable all the time. If I see something someone else has that I want, I make a plan for earning it myself and then implement that plan.

Every soul on Earth has their own issues and "stuff" they're working through. Until we walk a mile in their shoes, we should never say they have it better, or are better, than we are. If there's something we don't like about ourselves (and I think everyone has SOMETHING), we can step up and change it. If it's something that can't be changed, we can change our perception about it. It all starts with making a choice, and sticking with it.

Another nemesis of love and happiness involves grudges. Holding grudges because someone has hurt us, or made us angry, is an extremely liberating, and soul-freeing experience when its let go. Grudges are STIFLING. Anyone who's consciously released a grudge probably knows what I'm talking about. Not only do grudges create a bubble of negative energy around us, they're extremely stressful. Letting go of any and all grudges, and better yet embracing the person/s in that grudge emotionally, can change the entire dynamics of our lives. I don't mean we should go up to that person, give them a big ole hug, and say, "hey, I forgive you, even though you're a flipping jerk", we don't have to confront anyone we don't want to in order to forgive them. What I mean is by releasing the burden of the grudge from within ourselves, allows for forgiveness which is a pathway that can bring amazing personal contentment. The flipping jerk comment was just me kidding around.

Part of letting go of a grudge against someone, regardless of how much we think they're a jerk, is realizing that everyone on this planet is going through, or has gone through, something painful, or challenging. Whether it was a traumatic event from their childhood, or just having a rotten life in general, we must realize that not everyone deals with events or traumas in the same way, or with the same grace and acceptance as others. On occasion, sometimes, an event in one's life may turn that person into a very angry, intolerable person. Although this doesn't give anyone a free pass to treat someone else badly, in understanding and having empathy for that person, we can much easier shake off the misery they may have caused us. After all, it's unlikely it had anything to do with us in the first place.

Anger is another emotion that can be both dangerous, and healthy, depending on how it's utilized. I know I talk about me getting angry a lot, and it's true, I do. It's okay to get angry. It can be very motivating. However, getting angry to the point of turning various shades of red and raging and ranting, is probably not the best way to express it. Finding productive outlets to channel anger can be soul enriching and a powerful way to evoke change in whatever it is that makes us angry. Anger can encourage passion powerfully.

Our neighbors recently took the liberty of killing off a colony of bees on our property on the very day we were having them humanely removed. This action angered me to the point of action. I'm going to write an article on the importance of bees, and the future of a planet without them.

Cancer makes a lot of people angry.

After seeing so many people I care about die of colorectal cancer, I admit it made me very angry, too. Not just angry, but frustrated and powerless. I turned those emotions into determination, and threw myself even deeper into research and self-experimentation. Each death made me more determined to survive, and I was definitely going to show others that it could be done, as well.

Finding a space that is all ours, and only ours in this world is another sure way to happiness.

Creating a place where we can decorate it the way we want, and escape if we need to, can be another way of self-expression and happiness. A place where you can just hang out if you need to and be alone with your thoughts.

Having my own room at my Mother's with the color I chose on the walls and the furniture I wanted, and space for my favorite things, had made me very content. Last year she had the garage converted into an apartment for me, so now I have an even better place to escape to where I know I'm safe and can chill out in any way I choose.

Fortunately for me, medical marijuana is legal in California and I used it a lot in the early days living with

176

my grandmother. It was one of the only ways to control my bowel issues, tailbone pain, and the only way I could sleep on those rough nights. I wasn't comfortable smoking it inside my grandmother's house after the caregiver moved in because it bothered her. Even when I was locked up in my room with the window wide open, she could still smell it.

I would go outside to smoke when I could, but late at night, or when bathroom issues were at an all-time high, it was too difficult to go outside. As a result, I would go without it some nights when I really needed it. Privacy has always been an issue with my bathroom problems. I've grown used to not having it at the most critical moments, but now that I don't have that issue, I can see how important having privacy or a private retreat is in healing.

I like making lists of the things that bring happiness. Whether they're lists of things to do tomorrow, or of things to do a year from now. I've mentioned lists before, and I'll make another reference to them here. They can be useful in so many ways.

I keep a miniature notebook in my purse and only take it out to write in it, or to check it while in the store. I use it to make grocery lists, to-do lists, and even long term goal lists. I used it to remind myself of suggestions for this book. Without lists, my life would be a jumble of forgetful things. Get in the habit of making lists for organizational purposes. Nothing can free the mind more than feeling like you're not forgetting something all the time.

I added the chapter of Love and Happiness as a new chapter rather than incorporating it into the previous chapter because I believe love is a very important contributor to happiness that deserves special attention, as do the many facets of emotions and behaviors that can damage it.

The last thing I want to mention before closing out this chapter is a quality I was most guilty of, and one I believe can be a direct contributor to illness and disharmony. For lack of a better word, it's simply being "uptight". Some would refer to this as "anal retentive", or "fussy", or maybe even "high-strung."

I can honestly say I was an "uptight" person before my cancer diagnosis. I liked certain things to be a certain way, and if they weren't, I'd either have a fit about it, or just be angry about it. This is not a healthy way to be and if there's a cure for it, I would have to say that cure for me was cancer. I take things much slower these days, and if something goes awry with my plans about how something should be, I just change the way I think it should be. I don't get offended by most things that used to offend me anymore, and I'm usually able to laugh at myself when I make a mistake rather than bashing myself for it. I've learned how to relax and enjoy life rather than judge it and complain about it.

We're all capable of being beacons of love.

When we learn to appreciate each other along with our individual challenges whatever they may be, we're spreading love. When we accept people as what they are; just people, and when we are able to feel empathy for others, even those who have done us wrong, we're spreading love. When we understand our self-worth, and believe that everyone, including those with a deadly disease deserve love, we become open to love entering our lives. When we positively elevate our own behaviors and attitudes towards others, a contagious event takes place

178

where we might find ourselves smiling at strangers we pass on the street, or possibly getting urges to help someone get an item off a shelf they can't reach in the store. We become a person who spreads love everywhere we go, and therefore contribute to the happiness of other people. That in turn will increase our own happiness, well-being, and overall health.

15.
Chemotherapy and Western Medicine

The information about chemotherapy and Western medicine's methods for treating people with cancer is as numerous as it is controversial, no matter which cancer it is, or in what stage it's in.

Like I mentioned in a previous chapter, whether it works, or not, is debatable, but the one thing that everyone can agree on universally is that it is horrendously damaging to the body.

I'm not exactly sure how I know which damages to my body were caused by which treatment methods I experienced since each one of my doctors blamed the other one's treatments for the problems.

My radiation oncologist blamed the chemo for my osteoporosis, but I know it was from the radiation. I've heard of it happening to other people with even more devastating results than what happened to me. My bone pain started soon after the radiation treatments began.

The chemo caused many problems that my medical oncologist blamed the radiation for. My surgeon blamed the stricture on the radiation, but the part of my colon that was irradiated was removed by her, so I think it was the surgery that caused that.

The chemo made my skin light sensitive, and I still burn very easily when exposed to the sun, but I also tan after that burn, which I see as a benefit. It caused neuropathy in my legs and salivary glands that seems to be a permanent part of me now. It gave me chemo-brain, where I find it hard to remember names and numbers, something I had always been good at previously. I also get turned around in familiar areas on occasion, which had never happened to me in my life until during and after chemo. My short term memory has suffered as a result of chemotherapy, and sometimes I can't remember what someone told me not two minutes earlier. I'm sorry, did I already mention that? I even lost the ability to write. I don't mean physically, but mentally.

Writing has been my number one passion in life since I was four years old. It's been like a companion I can tell my most crazy ideas to, since my brain is constantly flooded with random stories that never happened and it was always my goal to someday publish an entire book, or two, or....

I realized I'd lost the ability to write when I sat down in 2009 to begin work on a story idea I'd had since I was ten years old.

The words were there in my head, but as soon as I started typing them, I either couldn't remember them, or I forgot that I already had written them not two minutes earlier.

It was the most frustrating, scary, and sad part of my whole experience thus far. What could I do if I couldn't write anymore? I thought I'd just have to die! Since I couldn't let that happen, I started writing the book anyway.

It was an unimaginable struggle that was probably a pretty shoddy piece of work, but I forced myself to just sit down and type, type, type.

Within a few months I was 500 pages into it and proud of myself for getting that far. I knew I'd have a hard time with the second and third drafts since I could hardly remember what happened on page ten, let alone page 510. I didn't worry about that and just kept on writing.

When it came to ending the book, I found I was unable to do it.

It just wasn't there.

I wracked my brain for four years trying to come up with an ending, but it just wouldn't come to me.

In the meantime, I started writing other books, including this one. I found this one was even harder to do. I thought it would be easier since the story was already there, but writing about real events is completely different from making ones up.

But it got easier as time went on. The ability was coming back slowly, but it was happening.

I can sit here and readily admit that chemotherapy definitely damaged my brain and I know it's still damaged by it, however, it has regained some old functions I thought were lost for good. I can remember ten digit numbers again after seeing them only once; especially if there are letters in them, but it's not completely reliable yet. As far as writing goes, with a lot of practice, writing became easy again.

When I was ready to begin work on the novel I started in 2009, I was unable to recover it because the program I'd used was incompatible with the new software of the times. I was as bummed as you could imagine, but I didn't let it deter me. I sat down and rewrote it to the best of my memory within three months, and surprisingly, the ending came to me and I was able to finish it. I published it in 2014 along with a short story compilation, and in 2015, I published my second novel.

As bad as some of the effects have been, I don't regret for a single moment doing any of the standardized treatments I did. The radiation/5FU shrank my tumor and allowed me to keep half of my rectum. It also irradiated the tumor and killed it.

I think it's very important not to regret our decisions, no matter what they are. I've said it before, and it's worth mentioning again and again, that a decision can always be changed to something else later on. The process of ridding ourselves of our unsolicited teacher (cancer) is going to be trial and error, for some of us, anyway.

When I solicited literary agents before publishing this book, I had one tell me he couldn't bear to read my cancer book because his father died of colorectal cancer and it would be too painful for him.

I can only imagine that loved ones finding out there are more productive ways to treat a disease after the fact could cause a lot of unnecessary guilt. It would be the same as if science found a cure the day after the loved one passed away. There isn't going to be any comfort in either of those instances, and in both instances, nothing would have changed the outcome.

For me, continuing chemotherapy after the first recurrence was not the correct answer. If the cancer ever comes back, I try everything in my arsenal before I'll do chemo again. That doesn't mean that it isn't for someone else. Belief in our treatments is an important part of them working, no matter what they are, as I mentioned in a previous chapter. There's a lot of information out there about chemo, and I will list references in the appendix on places to get more information. The best advice anyone can give is to get as much information as you can about your treatments; particularly the long term effects and particularly stories from other people who've done it. Talk to those who didn't do it, too, if you can find them, no matter what stage their cancer was in, but especially those with stage IV. There isn't many of us out there, especially those like me who didn't do chemo after having recurrences, or those who passed on chemo even though they were inoperable, but I know there are more of us out there, scattered about, keeping their silence. I can understand why, and I'll talk about that in a minute.

It wasn't easy for me to say no to chemo when all the experts were telling me it was my best chance for survival. It made my blood run cold each time I said no, wondering if they were really right. Even after the lung surgery when I knew chemo wouldn't work, there was an entire minute when I considered taking it just because of all the scary things the doctor was telling to me. Now I know for certain chemo was not my best chance for survival.

Just become informed. It seems to me that the people most likely to survive are the ones who researched every avenue to the tenth degree, and made their treatment decision fully informed. Don't be afraid to question doctors, either. If a doctor gives any attitude about being questioned or by being made accountable for their recommendations, it's definitely time to find another doctor.

I've tried to include as many suggestions, ideas and tools as I could, but I have no doubt there are many more available.

If chemo is chosen, I would try to compliment it with healthful alternatives such as acupuncture and massage therapy just to make myself feel emotionally healthier, if not physically better. One of my most important ingredients to my healing was happiness through contentment, and chemo treatments definitely weren't conducive to the success of that. Doesn't mean they won't be for someone else. I personally know people who've gone that route, but in all honesty, I've never seen that cure anyone. It just seems to help with symptoms.

My first oncologist wouldn't let me do antioxidants because he said they would counter the effects of the chemo. Healthy eating and juicing can still be done while on chemo if you can force yourself to eat. I recommend using TCM (Traditional Chinese Medicine) while doing chemo, if possible and I know people who've had great success using TCM alone. They can give you herb teas and acupuncture that helped me immensely after I did chemo. I listed a resource in the back of the book on how to find one, but the best way to find a TCM doctor, is to get recommendations from real people who've done it.

I have back-up plans for if I ever get another recurrence that's inoperable. I've always had back-up plans, and just having these plans made each recurrence that much easier to deal with. I had the plan, and I implemented it as soon as the grief and shock of the recurrence wore off. I've tweaked my back-up plans now that I've successfully cured a met with diet.

Anyone can decide not to do chemo and let nature do as it will. There is just as good a chance that someone who doesn't choose chemo will survive their cancer, as one who chooses chemo. As my oncologist told me, "there is no evidence either way whether chemo works, or not." Be-that-as-it-may, I believe doing nothing at all is a crap shoot. I've heard of people who claim they willed their cancer away and I'm not in any position to doubt them. But why not tilt the scales and make the survival odds much, much higher by whatever means necessary? By implementing a healthy diet, exercising in whatever way you can, practicing happiness, AND believing...

After my lung removal, I moved out of my stressful living arrangement, began taking enzymes, and devoted the majority of my time doing things that brought me joy. The plan worked brilliantly until another high-stress event occurred. Now that I've rid myself of that, I'm back on my happiness plan!

IF I get another recurrence, it will be surgery, and another diet change-up, more meditation and supplementing, and possibly a stay at an alternative treatment clinic that does hydrogen peroxide therapy, or concentrated juicing if the raw diet doesn't work. I'm not worried about that happening.

The Gerson clinic has been my plan C since I first found out about them early on in my cancer adventure. Plan C was if I ever became inoperable.

I have read and seen documentaries on The Gerson Method, and I'm more than convinced their method works. I know people personally who have used this method, and cured their cancer. One woman I know who was a stage III, did the program at home, and she's been cancer-free for sixteen years. She never did an ounce of chemo, which is outside the standards of care for a stage III, and is considered cured!

With Gerson, It's a two year deal to follow at home, that must be followed religiously. Their success rate is incredibly high. What's two years compared to a lifetime? See my resources in the back of the book for details.

There is a two week stay at the clinic recommended so they can teach you and your caregiver how to do the program at home. This is especially important for those of us who have done chemotherapy since it isn't recommended to do the coffee enemas without doctor supervision. This is probably because of the dangerous detoxing effects of flushing the heavy metals from the liver.

There are other places and methods to check out. I will list as many resources as I'm aware of, and I'll even research more options so those interested can choose the best one for them.

I have a friend who cured her bone cancer doing oxygen therapy in Mexico. The clinic she used is gone, but there are others and even some doctors here in the U.S. who employ H_2O_2 therapy treatments. They can't legally claim it cures cancer, but those it has helped claim otherwise.

Many of these plan C options are very costly.

My plan A to achieve my plan C was to raise the money needed to go. Anyone can raise money for their own cancer treatments. It's not necessarily an easy thing to do, but not only can it be done, but it can be another step in self-empowerment. I've never needed to do it, but I know others who have and they were very successful with it.

The ways I'd raise money is by selling my stuff online, doing garage sales, setting up for donations through online charity sites, and by applying for grants through the ACS and any other organization I can find that will help me. I've mentioned cancercare.org before. They gave me a little money in the beginning. There are online auction houses that can sell clothing, knick-knacks, and just about anything else. This is something anyone can do to raise money for their alternative treatments, no matter what they are and you don't necessarily have to be feeling super healthy to do it. All of this can be done online. If there are children in the family, raising money can be a really exciting project for them and take away some of the helpless feelings they might be experiencing.

Try not to be afraid to go this way if nothing else is working. Western doctors can only do so much and they're tremendously limited on what they can say and recommend, as well as with their knowledge on alternative choices. We can't expect them to cure us, only to help guide us toward available options, and even then, their options are limited to the restraints of their licensing. There are thousands of other options the doctors cannot tell you about, even if they wanted to. Some I've mentioned in here. Others are out there. Design your own. Take the control right out of cancer's hands. YOU CAN SURVIVE. You can. It's just up to you.

I want to take the time here to say I in no way believe our doctors are trying to kill us, as some who are against traditional treatments have claimed. Having spent five years of my disease with my first oncologist, I have no doubt he thought he was saving my life by pushing chemo. THIS IS WHAT HE WAS TRAINED TO DO. Doctors are products of their education and therefore he couldn't offer me any other options besides the protocol he was taught to give me. Luckily I am not a doctor and don't have to be held to such constraints. When I first began learning about all the people who were curing themselves, I was a little freaked out about why this information wasn't mainstream. If so many people are beating cancer without chemo, why aren't they plastering this information all over the news?

I've since learned why this is, and it's not just one reason.

For one thing, there is a credibility factor.

Being an advocate for going it without chemo, I've been moderately vocal about alternatives in my cancer groups and to other cancerians I've met who find out my history. The first thing they all want to know is how I've survived for so long? As soon as I tell them it's because I'm not doing chemo, I begin to lose them. Sometimes, they get downright defensive about it, as I've said. Some people start quoting chemo studies (not understanding the difference between relative numbers, and absolute ones). I can only imagine that these people feel like they've made bad choices in their own treatment plan and are lashing out at those of us who didn't, or maybe they watched a loved one suffer from the effects of chemo, and it's just too painful for them to think that person might have lived had they made another choice, like the literary agent who wouldn't consider this book. All I know for sure is that the information isn't getting mainstream attention because there aren't a lot of people doing it who are speaking out about doing it. I've seen it happen to the people I mentioned a few chapters ago in the support groups who spoke out about alternative treatments. Many of them were brow-beat into the ground for it, and they eventually stopped posting or commenting on anything about 'alternative' medicine. Some disappeared from the groups altogether and their beautiful success stories were lost to those whose lives could have been saved by them. The bashing has happened to me, as well, many times, but if I'd let those people make my decisions for me, I'd be in the same place as them, or worse.

Credibility for non-traditional treatments has also been damaged by militants who claim conspiracies against the government and/or pharmaceutical companies. Yes, pharmaceuticals are big business. Whether or not it's a conspiracy, I don't know. It's true that I wasn't handed all the information about the chemotherapy they were giving me, but it certainly wasn't hidden information. With the advent of the Internet, there is hardly any excuse to not be informed. If there is any question about whether or not something read online is true, simply ask your doctor. My doctor didn't lie to me when I asked him whether the chemo they were giving me worked or not. Again, don't be afraid to ask the right questions.

Another reason alternate methods of treating illness isn't mainstream information is because of what I call the "science-head syndrome."

It goes hand in hand with the credibility factor in that there aren't any clinical research studies being conducted to prove alternative methods of curing cancer work; at least not in the U.S. where it's all about money. It's a bit of a conundrum, since there are plenty of research studies being done on whether or not chemotherapy cures cancer, and even though science has NOT proven that chemo works, they use it anyway. The numbers used in those clinical research studies, and the way in which they're "worded" are not easily understood by people who can't speak mathematical statistics. I'm for sure one of them. However, I did take the time to learn a bit about how the numbers are calculated and reported in a research paper, and surprisingly, there is a very honest way to lie when dealing with statistics.

I'll say it again; science can't explain everything. In fact, I believe there is very little that science can accurately explain when dealing with the human body. With that, there doesn't seem to be any law that can't be broken.

Needing a research study to prove something is fact, is science-head mentality. That may not be a bad thing in some cases, but it could be a crippling thing when options are running out, and so is time.

Put cancer in a petri dish with chemo, and chemo most likely will kill it. Put cancer in a petri dish with bleach, and bleach will most likely kill it. Putting either of those cancer killers inside the body, and they may or may not kill the cancer. They also may or may not kill the patient! The only reason why research studies aren't being done on any alternative methods of killing cancer is simple. First of all, it costs money to conduct a clinical trial, and secondly, there is zero return on that money if the cure is something anyone can pull out of their garden or buy at their local supermarket. That's not a conspiracy. That's basic economics.

The doctors can't explain why I'm cancer-free. How could they? There's no research studies going on to find out why, and strangely enough, no one is breaking down my door to conduct scientific experiments on me to see what's different about me from every other person with colorectal cancer. They're not doing that to the ones who survive after so many chemo treatments, either. There simply isn't just one way to cure cancer that Western medicine has discovered. There may never be just one way to cure it, because it is such an individualized disease with so many individualized reasons for getting it. But when you look at what cancer is and the reasons behind why the human body's defenses can't destroy it, you can almost visualize what the problem is.

It brings me back to my introduction; cancer is the body's own cells going mutant and malignant. Since they're our own cells, our healthy cells think they're one of them and can't distinguish themselves from the malignant cells. Therefore they do nothing to destroy them. So what if we could teach our healthy cells how to distinguish themselves from a cancer cell? If we could do that, it's game over for the cancer cells. Well, we CAN do that! Quite simply we can turn our healthy cells into super-healthy cells where their appearance to the cancer cell is markedly different. That's what I imagine boosting the immune system with optimum nutrition does.

I did not allow the good opinion of others to scare me out of my decision to opt out of chemo treatments. It is a controversial road with very little support, but plenty of harsh criticism. There were a lot of people telling me I couldn't do it, but guess what? They're not saying that anymore.

I have a Facebook page in support of this book and its contents that I intend to keep very close tabs on. I will happily offer my support to those independent warriors walking the unpaved road. I also welcome anyone to the page who is doing traditional treatments to join our conversations. I will support anyone in any treatment regime they choose. The only discussions I will not tolerate on my page are haters that bash ANYONE for their treatment choices. The point to all of this is to heal

from our cancer in any way we can. Finding our own way
through this journey is very personal, but that doesn't
mean we can't help and guide each other through it
positively.

16.
A Matter of Raw Importance

When revising this book, I believe it's appropriate for me to add a chapter on the raw diet and its significance in the fight against cancer.

The first image that comes to many people's minds when you tell them you only eat raw food, are giant bowls of salads three times per day with an apple or pear thrown in on occasion.

It could be like that, if that's what someone preferred, but it is truly much more than that.

Having two, basic kitchen appliances can turn that image of continual salad eating into lasagna, corn chips, coconut cream pie, chocolate bars, and so much more.

When I was first introduced to the diet through my friend Aaron, and his friend Michelle; a raw food chef, I was blown away by the possibilities and even more by the rich and savory flavors the food afforded.

We spent hours preparing, experimenting, and eating everything we could in the raw repertoire.

Back then (the mid-nineties), we didn't have a high-powered blender or dehydrator to make the gourmet meals, so everything had to be hand crushed or air dried and though they were still yummy meals, it much more difficult to make the raw cheeses and chips that I adored.

Now I have a high-powered blender and a dehydrator, and making these gourmet meals is EASY.

I have dozens of books for raw food recipes, but nowadays, you can type anything you want into the computer, and at least one recipe will pop up for it. Want pizza? There are raw recipes for that. Want raw chocolate cake? There is that, too.

The most incredible thing about the raw diet that many think would be the complete opposite is the flavor of these foods. They don't have to marry to be delectable, but when they are, it's amazing!

Though the diet may not be for everyone over the long term, there simply isn't a better or faster way to improve our health than using the raw diet. My colon metastasis disappeared in as little as five weeks. Bigger problems might take longer, I don't know, but I recommend everyone give it a whirl for as long as I did it and see what it does to them.

You don't have to have the kitchen appliances I have to do the raw diet. It can be done much simpler if that's what you prefer, or if you get tired of doing a lot of preparation for the gourmet meals. Those are the recipes I'll list here. If you want something more complete, I can recommend getting a un-cook book from the Boutenko family. I have a couple of their books and they're simply experts at making just about any type of food raw. Their personal stories are quite remarkable, as well. My favorite un-cookbook by them was actually written by their kids. It's called, *Eating without Heating,* and that's where I got the raw corn chips recipe I use constantly even when I'm not doing my 99% raw diet.

Along with the corn chips I eat raw salsa. I make a big bowl of it that will last a week in the fridge and it's very basic to make. Three organic tomatoes, half a green bell-pepper (or red, if you prefer, or both if you prefer), half a yellow onion (or less, if you prefer), half a jalepeno (or less, if you prefer), a half bunch of organic cilantro, a tablespoon of cold-pressed olive oil, a pinch of salt and pepper, two or three diced cloves of garlic. If you want to put a twist on it, you can add half of a diced orange to it. I have to admit, I practically lived on the chips and salsa it was soooo good!

If you like to juice, and I do while I'm raw, I juice the vegetables first and separate the pulp before I juice the fruit. Then I use the vegetable pulp to make garden burgers.

I simply but it in a food processor or blender and add a little flaxmeal and olive oil to it so it will bunch up and stick together. I form them into patties, and dehydrate them for five to ten hours. That makes enough patties for a few days, at least.

I use the garden patties in sandwiches of sprouted bread (not 100% raw, so that's where the 99% raw comes in), some mustard or cold-pressed vegenaise, some raw hummus, a slice of tomato, onion, and a small wedge of lettuce.

There are raw dairy cheeses available in certain places that I used very sparingly while on the diet. I wouldn't recommend them since I didn't use them when I cleared up the met, so just FYI on that.

Another thing I like to eat while on the raw diet is marinated mushrooms. I just soak them in a little Nama Shoyu or Tamari (these are similar to soy sauce but prepared raw; Nama Shoyu, or with low heat). Soak them for a few hours and they become lightly cooked.

You can cook anything using the sun on the raw diet. I

knew someone once who had strings and strings with tomatoes and other fruits and veggies pinned to them in the windows of his house. I prefer using mason jars for sun drying. To make sun-dried tomatoes, you have to use a jar because you need to soak them in olive oil.

If you only get one thing for your raw kitchen, I recommend you choose a high-powered blender. For a top-of-the-line one, you can pay anywhere from $300-$400 dollars, but there are sufficient ones that cost less than half that amount. The one I use is the Ninja. If you want to make your own nut-butters and cheeses, this is the only way to go. Using anything less than a powered machine and it takes hours to make just a little bit. Yes, I learned this the hard way.

To make your own almond or cashew milk, nothing high-powered is required, but you'll get more bang for your buck with a high-powered machine.

As most of us in life live on tight budgets, I got most of my equipment used online. The Champion Juicer (the one I think is the best), costs a couple hundred dollars new. I paid around $70 for my used one in 2009, and it still works like a Champ! My dehydrator was also purchased used for about $30, and it's one of the large, circular ones that have tiered trays. I bought it years ago, and though it's really old, the company still sells replacement trays for it. It came with about four trays and I've since added three more. As far as my high-powered blender...my sweet brother and his wife got me one for Christmas one year, so I lucked out there!

A dehydrator is a very, very nice thing to have, especially when you're raw. You can just do so much with it. I get what I call 'the crunchies' if I go too long without

197

something crunchy to eat. I know other people that get the crunchies, too, if they've been juicing for a long time, or doing liquid diets. I think it comes from having food addictions, but I'm not certain about that. All I know is that if I don't have something crackery crunchy after a while I start to feel deprived.

The dehydrator can make all kinds of crunchy raw foods like crackers, chips, peanut brittle, pizza…and it's all still considered raw because it's slow cooked on very low temperatures that don't destroy the nutrients in the food. I never dehydrate anything above 105 degrees F, but I you could go higher and still preserve the food.

One of the best things about the raw diet is all the healthy oils, avocados and nuts you can have and they won't be unhealthy: Unless of course that's all you're eating. Be sure to have a wide variety of fruits and vegetables. I tend to find a few things I like and get trapped just eating those things. That's probably one of the reasons I can't tolerate the diet for as long as I'd like to.

One last thing about the raw diet; there are now companies that specialize in packaged raw foods. There are whole meals and snacks available, for a price. The Squeeze, out of New York makes the most heavenly peanut brittle. I figured out how to make it myself in my dehydrator, but if you're pressed for time, and really want something that takes hours to dehydrate, most health food stores carry a line of raw food and snacks.

17.
FOUNDATION STRONG;
I'm a Brick House

Every day I practice building the strengths of my formula. Even though I'm currently cancer-free, I never take it for granted.

I may eat something I shouldn't, or some other thing that isn't necessarily healthy for me once in a while, but when I do, I'm very mindful that that behavior isn't going to become a habit. Part of my happiness stems by not always following the rules. My foundation is strong, and the tools I need to stay healthy are ALWAYS in the forefront of my mind and I utilize them daily.

I have a very strong feeling that my cancer is gone for good. The reality is that it could very well show up again, or that even a new one could arise someday. That will be a possibility for the rest of my life. However, I feel in the pursuit of my personal cure, I've given myself the knowledge I need to conquer it again if it ever does come back and I don't spend my life worrying about it. A new plan is all it will take, and there is no doubt anywhere in my being that I couldn't beat it back down again if need be and maintain the high quality of my life.

In writing this memoir, I was well aware that there may be some backlash from nay-sayers who don't believe the suggestions I've talked about here-in, just like the people I have run across in the support groups. All I can do is repeat to them what I just said in the last chapter. I wouldn't be where I am today, healthy, happy, and cancer-free, if I'd listened to them instead of following my own way. I never let the nay-sayers scare me into making decisions that they thought were best, and THAT was my foundation. There will always be nay-sayers trying to tell us we can't do something just because they can't, or won't. If you want to rub your left thumb with your right index finger because it worked on someone else's cancer and it feels right for you, you go right ahead and do it! I have never lost my resolve to cure myself, no matter what anyone else had to say about it.

There may also be some who are critical of the term cancer survivor, or cancer warrior to describe someone with cancer. To me it in no way implies that I was ever a victim or that cancer was an enemy that I was at war with. To me, the terms are a descriptive example of the soul and determination it takes for an individual to face the daunting challenges cancer creates and come out of it for the better.

My cancer has left an indelible imprint on my body and on my life. I will forever be in some sort of pain or other, whether it's from the fractured tailbone, the bothersome stricture, or the neuropathy, but I still plan someday on doing either a mud run, or a triathlon, or both!

My cancer has freed me from nearly every fear and phobia I had. Without fear crippling and sabotaging me, I've been able to pursue my professional dream of having the books I've written over the years, published, starting with this one, the most important. Before my cancer journey I was terrified to let another person read my writings. My lifelong, debilitating fear of heights has apparently vanished, too.

I love my cancer. If that simple statement is offensive to those who hear it, it's only because they haven't developed the relationship with cancer that I have. Cancer is, and always will be, a huge part of me. Saying I hate cancer is the same as saying I hate myself, and that in no way describes me. I love myself, and I let the words I say, and the words in my internal mind reflect that feeling every day.

Thank you, cancer, for coming into my life, slapping me around a bit to wake me up, then periodically vanishing into thin air. I have your heavy footprints to remind me of our time together, and although you won't be missed, you will never be forgotten. Good point and Good-bye.

Maximus magister.

Come visit me on the book's facebook page. All visitors are welcome!

https://www.facebook.com/MetastaticColorectalCancer?ref=hl

Epilogue;
A Semicolon Among Colons

I first heard the term "Semicolon" to describe those who've had colon resection surgery on my online colorectal cancer board. It was a term going around there years before I ever arrived.

The term isn't just a clever pun for those who are missing parts of their colon. For me, it explains the essence of my existence. With the daily, hourly, and sometimes minute by minute bathroom issues I contend with, I'm reminded constantly that I'm missing a portion of my colon and my body will never function as it did with a "full" colon again.

The term has another meaning for me though, too.

The definition of a semicolon is having a closer relationship to the last clause than a comma can do. Like a long pause, or for putting emphasis on the latter sentence.

A colon, on the other hand, marks the end of the clause: A continuance, but still the end.

The meaning of being a semicolon for me is that the story, my story, is continuing. I'm missing part of my colon, but...I'm surviving. I'm here, sharing my story; living proof that our own bodies CAN fight off a terminal illness. It's not only possible to survive stage IV colorectal cancer outside the traditional standards of care, but by working with, and figuring out our bodies and giving them the tools they need to do so, it's definitely probable.

Every "incurable" disease I was diagnosed with is now nonexistent in my body, save the neuropathy. The cancer is gone, the diabetes is gone…I'm not in a wheelchair, and I don't need to take any osteoporosis medications. I didn't have my tailbone cemented as the doctors wanted to do, and I manage my pain with non-debilitating meditation when I have to, and breathing exercises. It's definitely not perfect, but I'm managing my life as I see fit and it can hardly get better than that. I took control of my disease, instead of letting my disease control me. I did that by researching both my disease, and my own body. One I did online and through books, the other through trial, error, and self-analysis.

I made my body and mind a hostile environment for cancer.

Cancer is an anaerobic organism that cannot survive in an oxygen rich environment. Perfect! I flooded my body with oxygen by exercising regularly, and using deep breathing techniques.

Cancer doesn't like a strong immune system, either, so I ate healthy and incorporated superfoods and antioxidants into my diet.

I believe that heavy, genuine laughter strengthens the immune system, too. I've cracked ribs laughing, and thought I'd split my spleen on more than one occasion simply by enjoying a funny joke! I make it a point to spend as much time as I can with the two people who make me laugh the hardest; my nephew, Gage, and my bud, Aaron. I laugh a lot with all of my friends and family. My three best girlfriends make me laugh, too. Susan, Crystal, and my girl Monkey who used to kill me with laughter! Too bad the Monk lives so far away now.

There is definitely a cure for colorectal cancer, many, in fact. If there wasn't, it would have a 100% mortality rate, and it doesn't. It is my greatest hope that my story and suggestions inspire those who read it and that they too, find their own personal pathway to healing and to a cure. It's within us all and we all deserve to have it.

August 7th, 2013.

Time moves in slow motion.

I find myself sitting on the edge of the bed, staring off into nothing. I go to the closet and rummage around in my pink fabric box for the cough medicine from last cold season. I find a twin package of specially sized light bulbs with only one bulb left in the package. Months earlier I had been tearing up my room looking for that very package when the bulb died in my small, Tiffany-style lamp that I absolutely adore. What luck to find that package now!

I take a huge swig of the cough medicine. The gooey red liquid instantly coats my throat and stomach with the comforting warmth of false security. I take another swig for good measure, and dig the light bulb out from its half secure location in the flimsy plastic packaging. Half expecting the bulb to not fit, I screw it into the Tiffany-style lamp that rests in my wicker bookcase; exactly across the room from the bed. I click the switch, and the beautiful purple, red and blue rectangular panes of stained glass with the dragonflies all around it, illuminates the room that had previously been lit by only two small candles.

I go back and sit on the edge of the bed, staring at the lamp. Memories of when my grandmother gave me the lamp play havoc in my head. Which birthday was it? Or was it a Christmas gift? Seems like it was just one of those times when she gave me a gift simply because she loved me. She had been known to do things like that from time to time. Maybe when she first saw the lamp in the store she anticipated subconsciously that this very moment would someday occur so she bought it on a whim not really knowing why. Whatever the reason, it didn't matter. The only thing that mattered now was that it was from her, and more than ever before, I really needed that lamp.

The warmth of the cough medicine was wearing off. I'm still not asleep and it's pushing 2 am. I go to the closet and take yet another tasty swig. Instantly warm again. I ask myself the stupid question of whether or not I was self-medicating, and begin wondering how much cough syrup was too much. Could I actually overdose on this stuff? I laugh at my irrelevant questioning of myself. Was that a genuine laugh coming out of me? I wish I had a cigarette, but dammit...I quit smoking a year and a half ago. Still, I wish I had a cigarette.

I'm wearing a dent in the edge of the bed. Better get up and get more cough syrup. Eventually I must get sleepy, yes...eventually?

I must take enough cough medicine to prevent me from dreaming. Dreaming was the worst thing that could happen right now. I must not sleep if I have to dream.

So I stare numbly at the little Tiffany-style lamp that my grandmother gave me some years ago, and ponder the reasons why, after so many months of looking, I find the light bulb to that lamp, tonight, of all nights, and so easily?

My red and puffy eyes tell the tale of the experiences of

the day. My grandmother, after several years of a painfully slow decline in health, died peacefully with half of her family at her side tonight. My Mother, my aunt, my niece and I, standing around her, letting her know we thought it was okay for her to let go and join her loved ones who had passed before her. Four generations represented on this night, gently petting her as she slipped away. Twenty-two days before her 91st birthday, and fifteen hours before the last of her fourth generation was born. A very long and full life, yes. How fortunate was I, and the rest of my family, to have her here for that many years! Her lifespan was over, but that didn't mean I wasn't going to miss her for the rest of my life. It didn't mean I wasn't going to heavily feel like something, or someone very special was missing from every single important or insignificant life event that occurred to me from here on out.

My grandmother had great belief in me. She encouraged me to keep up my writing and actually enjoyed my crazy musings. I would find scraps of paper with my stories on them tucked in various places around her house, all the time. She saved everything I ever wrote; most of it things I hadn't even remembered creating, some of it from when I was too young to even know the whole alphabet yet.

A writer and skilled researcher herself, she wrote two books on genealogy, spending years compiling information on two separate family trees. She was a daughter of the American Revolution, and a member of the third order of the Franciscan Catholic Church. She was a self-trained carpenter, successful family cook, and the Matriarch of her family for the fifty years after her husband passed away.

For me, my grandmother was my nurturer and I had always looked forward to staying the night with her as a child. We had our routine of the shows we would watch; The Love Boat, Fantasy Island, and Quincy Jones, M.D., and all the yummy cookies we would bake. Then she would cuddle with me on the couch and make me feel like all was safe and right in the world. The security she gave me didn't end when I grew up. As my brother says, "Mama was our rock."

So as I sit silently on the edge of the bed, looking in the direction of the small, Tiffany-style lamp glowing peacefully from the wicker bookcase, my vision begins to blur. The cough medicine is definitely kicking in. My swollen eyes are getting heavy and I can feel my heart rate slowing down to a mercifully normal beat.

Tomorrow is the first day I must start living without my loving grandmother in the world. I don't know yet how I'm going to do that...If it's even possible I can do that...

I love you so much, dear, sweet, Mama. Your memory lives on in my heart, as your presence is forever in my soul.

R.I.P.
Alice Daniel Pritchard
August 29, 1922 - August 7, 2013

https://www.youtube.com/watch?v=JHEBzxAV5f4

APPENDIX

i.

CANCER-ESA-PEAS

Here are some recipes designed to both nourish healthy cells, and kill cancer cells. For the revised edition (2nd edition) of this book, I've added a couple raw recipes besides the ones listed in the raw chapter. To me, the raw diet is the optimum one for kicking cancer's rear-end. The more raw, organic fruits and vegetables a person can add to their diet, the more pure nutrition they're going to get.

Cancer killers are foods that I add to at least one meal per day, every day. No matter what I eat, I find I can add these simple foods to it. I even sometimes carry a small plastic container around with me with these foods in them, already prepared, and ready to add to whatever I eat on the go.

1.   BROCCOLI is one of the most important and easy to add foods that everyone should eat regularly. Lightly steamed till bright green: Broccoli is one of the most helpful cancer defeating foods you can eat. Organic preferably.

2.   MUSHROOMS, especially specific species have been proven to have cancer destructive properties. Chaga, a bark-like mushroom that grows on the trunks of birch trees, is known in Chinese medicine as "The King of Herbs". It can be found in supplement form, or in teas from Chinese medicine doctors. Maitake mushrooms are also known to kill cancer. I add maitake and/or shiitake mushrooms to most of my food, cooked. I have heard that mushrooms need to be cooked in order for us to assimilate their usefulness. Lightly steamed should be sufficient. I have read that mushrooms are one of the foods that should especially be organic, but they are usually very costly to get that way. I have found organic maiitake's in my area that are affordable, but mostly I buy from Asian markets that have dried shiitake. I believe the benefit of mushrooms is important enough to not be too concerned about whether or not they're organic.

3.   TURMERIC, and/or curry, is another one of my favorite tricks in defeating colorectal cancer. Turmeric is especially good for the intestines and intestinal tract. I add a pinch or more to every meal I cook.

4.   LEMONS are another food I add to everything. It started out with just enjoying the flavor, then a friend of mine sent me an article on how lemons defeat cancer. I don't know if they do, but a couple of thin slivers, peel, and all, added to food adds a tasty zest to every dish! I add slices to sandwich's, on top of sushi, and even little pieces in my spaghetti sauce.

5.   APPLES are full of sugar, which is sort of a conundrum when dealing with cancer. Not all sugars are alike, and for some reason I can't explain, some sugars do not seem to be harmful. When I discovered that cancer thrived on sugar, I tried very hard to eliminate sugar entirely from my diet. I found it was impossible. Especially being a vegetarian, which I was at the time. There were people who claimed to have cured their cancer juicing carrots and apples which are both very high in sugar, so I figure the nutritional value of the carrots and apples outweighed and over powered the feeding frenzy of the cancer. Whatever it is, I do like juicing apples and carrots, along with other things. When I'm not juicing, I love to grab an organic apple, and eat it right off the core. I believe the saying, "an apple a day keeps the doctor away".

2. APPLE CIDAR VINEGAR to me is a mystery healing agent. Vinegar doesn't appear to have much nutritional value, yet apple cidar vinegar is believed to have many healing properties, and I believe in it. As I've stated before, some things science just can't explain. I use apple cidar vinegar in recipes, in my home made raw dog food, and sometimes I just down a teaspoon of it, which is awful! It is a fermented food, so it is possible that it will help in adding probiotics to the intestines.

2. ALKALINE WATER & FOOD is another option, and I drink the water on occasion. There is a lot of information about the correlation between cancer

and a high acidic body. I definitely subscribe to this as a possible solution. It makes sense. There are machines that can control the pH of water, but they are very expensive right now for most of us. There are bottled waters sold at health food stores that have higher pH's, but they are pricey, too. I only drink them on occasion, and I prefer a 9.5 pH. The higher the pH, the more alkaline the water, with the highest possible number being 14, and a neutral number being seven. Our stomachs have a pH of about 2. Drink on an empty stomach ½ an hour before eating to avoid changing the pH in the stomach. PH levels in the body could arguably be raised by eating alkaline promoting foods, too. Here is a website to look at: http://www.webmd.com/diet/features/alkaline-diets-what-to-know. As I've mentioned before, doing research is very empowering.

The following recipes are designed to be simple, include my cancer fighting ingredients, and best of all, they're tasty!

Aside from adding certain things to our diets to stay healthy, we must eliminate some other things that feed, or promote cancer.

I mentioned the sugar factor.

We know sugar feeds cancer because one of the best diagnostic tools they use to diagnose cancer, the PET scan. It works by detecting cancer in the body by lighting up the area where the highest metabolic processing of sugar is happening...in other words, where a cancer smorgasborg is happening.

Processed foods are LOADED with sugar. Not just sugar, but high fructose corn syrup, evaporated cane juice, fructose, sucralose, and other hidden names...there is an ever growing list of sugars added to processed foods. I have no idea the need for food companies to add so much sweetening agents to EVERYTHING. All I know is to stay away from them. I read the labels on everything I buy. I've been doing it for so long, I pretty much know which brands do and don't add sugar. It's very good information to have if you want to buy something as simple as tomato sauce.

My best advice is to stay away from added sweeteners, be it natural, or otherwise. Artificial sweeteners are worse than refined sugars in many ways, and I avoid them even more strongly than I do refined sugar. Aspartame is one of the BIGGEST no-no's, ever.

I eat very little pre-packaged meals, and as I've noted before, I read the labels on everything. After doing this for a while, I know instinctively what's off my menu.

So here are some especially nummy-nummy cancer-esa-peas to appease the taste buds, and fuel our healthy cells! G=gluten-free, V=vegan, S=sugar-free, R=raw.

Easy Peasy Cheesy Casserole (G,V,S)

1 pkg wide rice noodles (or any wide wheat-free, wavy noodles)
¾ cup nutritional yeast flakes
1 cup soy, almond, or rice milk (plain, unsweetened)
2 tbs. Tahini

2 tbs. cornstarch
1 tsp. turmeric
1 tsp. garlic powder
1½ tsp. black pepper
a pinch cinnamon
1 tsp. agave or honey
½ tsp. sea salt, or pink Himalayan salt
2 thin slices of lemon with rind, chopped
2 cups chopped mushrooms of choice
1 ½ cup peas
One crown broccoli, washed and chopped
Half a bag of fake chicken strips (optional)

Boil noodles until soft, but al dente. Put aside.

In a sauce pan, combine the milk, tahini, agave, yeast, cornstarch, and spices with ½ tsp. pepper. Simmer until it starts to thicken. Add peas, fake chicken, mushrooms, and broccoli. Stir until broccoli is bright green (about three to five minutes). Remove from heat.

In a baking dish, add the noodles and sauce, and stir together until combined well, sprinkle the top with the rest of the pepper. Cover with lid, and put in the oven at 350 degrees for twenty to thirty minutes. Add the chopped lemon slices.

For an even cheesier version of this recipe for non-vegans, add a thin layer of low fat cheddar cheese to the top of the casserole just before putting it into the oven. Morning Star and Boca both make a version of fake chicken strips that can be bought at nearly any grocery store, including some Targets. They may change the meal to non-gluten-free, however. Some meat substitutes are gluten-free. Please check the appendix. I will list some.

Optimal Marinara (G,V,S)

1 can tomato sauce (no sugar added)
1 can diced tomato (no sugar added)
or
1 jar of spaghetti sauce (no sugar added)
½ onion, chopped
1 tsp. garlic powder, or 2 cloves, chopped
½ cup red wine (chianti) (optional)
2 tbs. basil
½ tsp. turmeric
pinch sea salt
1 tsp. pepper
pinch of cayenne
2 tbs. oregano
1 tbs. rosemary
1 bay leaf
1 tsp. agave or honey
pinch cinnamon
1 tsp. apple cider vinegar
1 zucchini, chopped (optional)
1 to 2 cups chopped mushrooms of choice
2 thin slices of lemon with rind, chopped

Combine all ingredients except the lemon in a saucepan, and simmer for fifteen or twenty minutes. Add lemon after cooking, and combine. Pour over any desired pasta.

Soyrizo Arroz (V)

2 cups rice uncooked
½ package soyrizo (veggie chorizo can be found
at health food stores, and Wal-mart)
1 cups mushrooms of choice
¼- ½ cup yellow onion diced
2-3 cloves garlic, minced
1 tsp. shallots (optional)
1 tsp. pepper
1 tsp. Celtic sea salt or pink Himalayan salt
2 thin slices lemon with zest, chopped
1-2 crown broccoli steamed

Cook the mushrooms with the rice until rice is tender and al dente. Add the soyrizo, onion, garlic and spices. Cook for about ten minutes, stirring occasionally. Take off the heat, and add the lemon. Eat with a side of broccoli and the below salad for a complete meal.

Cancer Killer Salad

With Chemo-less Dressing (G,V,S)

1 bowl of spring mix salad, organic
1 cup raw organic spinach
handful of organic grape tomatoes, or
a sliced up organic beefsteak tomato
lg pinch of pickled beets
lg pinch of sourkraut
three slices purple onion

½ sliced up carrot
3 broccoli florets
1 tbs. minced garlic
3 thinly sliced lemon with zest, cut in halves
Anything else that sounds good

Chemo-less Dressing (V,S)

2 tbs. tahini
1 cup light sodium soy sauce
(for gluten-free version, find wheat-free soy sauce)
1 large ripe avocado
1 tbs. cold pressed olive oil, or flaxseed oil
1 tsp. apple cider vinegar
½ tsp. turmeric
½ tsp. pepper
small pinch of cinnamon
1 tsp. minced garlic

Combine all ingredients of the dressing, and mix well. Pour as much over the cancer killer salad as you want, and enjoy!

Gluten-less Apple Cake (G, S)

1 ½ cups millet or rice flour
½ tsp stevia (optional)
1 tsp baking soda
½ tsp baking powder
1 tsp powdered cinnamon

1 medium banana
1 cup unsweetened applesauce
1 cup chopped apple of choice
six apple slices of choice
¾ cup plain greek yogurt, or fat free sour cream
2 tbs coconut oil

In a mixing bowl, mix the flour, baking soda, baking powder, stevia and cinnamon together well. Put aside.

In a different bowl, mix together the yogurt, banana, applesauce, chopped apples and oil.

Pour the yogurt mixture into the flour mixture, and combine. Add a little water, or almond milk, just enough to loosen the batter enough for stirring.

Spray a 9x9" baking pan with non-stick coconut spray, and pour the apple batter into it evenly. Place the six apple slices on top of the batter, fanning out from the center. Bake at 350 degrees until golden brown on top, and a toothpick runs smooth through the center. About 40 minutes.

Avocado Dressing (R, G, V, S)

1 hass or ½ reed avocado
1 cup Nama Shoyu or wheat-free, tamari
1 tsp. apple cider vinegar
2 tbs. cold-pressed olive oil
2 tbs. raw tahini (sesame butter)
pinch of Celtic sea salt & pepper

1 tsp. organic lemon juice

Mash the avocado and tahini together until they form a paste. Add all other ingredients and combine until smooth. Pour over salad or use as a dip for vegetables.

Sunflower Cheese Spread (G, V, S, R)

2 cups raw sunflower seeds
½ cup organic lemon juice
1 tsp. apple cider vinegar
½ tsp. lemon zest
2 tbs. raw tahini
2 sprigs parsley
1 tbs. olive oil
½ tsp. Celtic sea salt & pepper
2 cloves garlic
1 tbs. nutritional yeast flakes
½ tsp. agave or honey if not concerned about vegan

Soak the sunflower seeds overnight in pure water. Rinse the next morning letting the loose hulls of the seeds drain with the water if you can.
Blend in a high-powered blender or food processor along with the tahini, nutritional yeast flakes, and lemon zest until it starts to bulk up. When it does that, add first the lemon juice, garlic, and remaining ingredients. If it bulks up too much, add very small amounts of water being careful not to let it get runny. Use as a spread, cheese substitute, or dip.

ii.
Glossary

5-FU: Fluorourocel; is a chemotherapy agent that has been in use for about 40 years. Often used in conjunction with radiation as a pre-adjuvant chemo.

Adhesions: Tissue that forms and connects two different tissues together, such as the abdominal wall connecting to the outside of the intestinal wall, caused by surgeries, inflammation, or injuries. The tissues can no longer move freely inside the body with adhesions causing pain.

Adjuvant Chemo: Chemotherapy treatment given after the initial, or primary treatment. Also known as "mop up" chemo. Given to patients who have no actively seen cancer, but intended to kill off any microscopic cancer cells that may still be in the body.

 Anastomotic Stricture: A narrowing of the colon wall caused by scarring following colon resection or laparoscopic gastric by-pass surgery.

Anemia: An abnormally low number of red blood cells, or hemoglobin inside the cells.

Anesthetize: To render unconscious or to otherwise desensitize an area with the use of pharmaceutical drugs.

CBC: Complete Blood Count. Typically used to see if red blood cells, white blood cells and platelets are within normal range. An abnormal blood count can indicate many types of problems.

CDC: Center for Disease Control and Prevention. A government agency that monitors, collects data, and reports on disease and illness. From their site: www.cdc.gov

Collaborating to create the expertise, information, and tools that people and communities need to protect their health – through health promotion, prevention of disease, injury and disability, and preparedness for new health threats.

CMS: In San Diego County, CMS is County Medical Services. They are a local government agency that isn't considered insurance, but will pay for emergency medical treatments and/or procedures for qualifying, low income persons. Other cities and counties may have similar services. For contact information for CMS, please refer to the resources section of the appendix.

CT/CAT Scan: Computed tomography/Computed Axial Tomography, is an x-ray that takes cross sectioned pictured of the inside of the body. Takes much clearer pictures than an actual x-ray, and can show organs, blood vessels, and other soft tissues.

Catheter: A flexible tube that goes into any orifice of the body meant to open up the passageways and to allow the natural flow of fluids to continue as normal. An example is a tube used to open up a blocked urethra so urine can flow again.

Centrifugal: Moving away from an axis. Centrifugal juicers spin and grind the food, separating the pulp from the juice.

Colonoscopy: A diagnostic procedure where the doctor places a flexible, long necked camera into the rectum, and can guide the camera up the colon to view the lining. There is a pronged arm attached to the camera that can take samples of any anomalies, or completely remove most polyps.

Colon Resection: The surgery that removes a portion of the colon, and reattaches the cut ends of the colon.

Colostomy: A surgical procedure where a part of the large intestine is sewn through a hole in the abdomen (stoma), where waste has an alternative route from the body. Can be reconnected under some conditions.

Conditioned Emotional Response: Is an event or action that often enough to induce the same emotional response each time the same event or action occurs.

Contrast: An intravenous or oral radiocontrast agent used to make contrasting images during certain body scans. The radiocontrast agent used during a PET scan is radioactive glucose.

Cystitis: Inflammation of the bladder. Can be caused by bacteria, or fungus, but can also be caused by radiation therapy, drugs, catheters, or as a complication from other diseases.

Demerol: An opioid analgesic, or painkiller. It can be given orally by prescription. Typically used as an anesthetic for conscious sedation during certain procedures, in conjunction with an amnesiac drug, or a drug that causes memory loss of the procedure.

Diagnosis: The mystery as to why we're sick is discovered and proved. Identity of symptoms revealed.

ER: Abbreviation for the Emergency Room of hospitals.

FOLFOX: Or FOLFOX 6 is a chemotherapy typically used for colorectal cancer patients as an adjuvant treatment. It consists of Oxaliplatin, and 5FU. It's usually given in two week increments for six to eight months.

GI: Abbreviation for a Gastroenterologist physician,

or Gastro-intestinal, or disorders of the gastrointestinal tract. Could also be short for Government issue, but that hardly pertains here.

Golytly/halflytly: The salty beverage used 24 hours prior to a GI procedure that cleans out and collapses the intestinal tract. Also known as bowel prep.

Hernia: A protrusion of an organ, or part of such organ that pokes through a weak spot in the wall of that organ.

Ileostomy: An ostomy that is from the small intestine, not the large.

Incontinence: The inability to hold back bodily functions such as urination or defecation.

Infusion: A way in which chemotherapy can be administered intravenously into a patient.

Insufficiency Fractures: Fractures caused when the bone isn't strong enough to support normal amounts of pressure. Can be caused by osteoporosis, radiation damage, or lack of nutrients in the diet.

Lesion: A change in tissue that is abnormal. Can happen anywhere in, or outside of the body.

MRI: Magnetic Resonance Imaging is a type of scan that uses magnets to get a more detailed viewing of the inside of the body than an x-ray can.

Malignant: Life threatening, diseased, cancerous.

Mass: Generally used to describe a tumor, or of an unknown collection of cells found in the body.

Medi-Cal: Medical insurance issued by California State government for persons under 21 years of age, or over 65 years of age who qualify, and for disabled persons receiving SSI.

Metastasis/Mets: A secondary cancer growth from the primary cancer site, to another part of the body. Generally indicating the stage a cancer is in. When spread from the primary site to another site, the stage is IV.

Mitosis: The rate at which a cell reproduces itself.

NED: The three best letters in the alphabet; No Evidence of Disease.

Neuropathy: Peripheral neuropathy is basically damage to the nervous system, in this case by chemotherapy. It can cause hot/cold sensitivity in just about any area of the body, but particularly to the hands and feet in most patients.

OBGYN: A physician specializing in women's studies, or obstetrics and gynecology.

Obstruction: A blockage in the intestines caused by waste build up, or a narrowing of the colon walls.

Oncology: The medical study of cancer.

Osteoporosis: A thinning of the bones. Changes in quality and density of the bone, possibly from calcium deficiencies, and/or age.

PICC Line: Peripherally inserted central catheter inserted into a vein for indefinite period of time. Used for patients in chemotherapy, similar to the portacath.

Porta-cath: Medical appliance implanted under the skin of the chest and into a vein in the neck for immediate administration of medicine. Patients receiving chemotherapy treatments often have one of these, or a PICC line.

Pre-adjuvant Chemo: A chemotherapy treatment or treatments used to shrink a tumor before it can be surgically removed.

Primary: Original cancer, or point where the original cancer began. For example: Cancer originating in the colon is colorectal cancer, where if the cancer spreads to the lungs, it is "primary colorectal cancer with metastasis to the lung." Lung cancer is a different cancer altogether.

Prognosis: The medical expected outcome of the disease.

Psychosomatics: The mind controlling the body.

Pulmonologist: A physician specializing in the respiratory tract, and lungs.

SSI: Supplemental Security Income. For disabled persons who do not qualify for SSA.

Spindly: Slender or spiky appearance. Elongated spines on a tumor indicates it could be cancerous.

Stool: A more pleasant word to describe feces, crap, sh*t, or poop.

Takedown Surgery: Surgery to reverse an ostomy.

Tumor: A fluid containing, or solid mass that appears abnormally where a mass shouldn't be. Can be inside or outside of the body. Can be malignant, or benign.

Versed: An amnesiac drug typically used for conscious sedation, so the patient doesn't remember the procedure.

Vitals: Vital signs are heart-rate, blood pressure, temperature, pulse rate, and respiration rate. Vitals are the first thing that's usually done at doctor appointments.

Zappings: The word I use to describe radiation treatments.

iii.

ORGANIC FOODS LIST

The following list is fruits and vegetables that should always be organic, or unsprayed.
As recommended by Dr. Andrew Weil

- Apples
- Strawberries
- Grapes
- Celery
- Peaches
- Spinach
- Sweet bell peppers
- Nectarines
- Cucumbers
- Potatoes
- Cherry tomatoes
- Hot peppers

Kale, collard greens, and summer squash are also recommended to be organic.

I think all thin skinned fruits and veggies should be organic or unsprayed, especially foods that don't have skins at all, such as lettuce.

Also, be sure you wash your fruits and vegetables before consuming. Some may argue that when washing our foods, all the minerals are being washed off of them, too. If this is a concern, then wash them lightly.

The importance of eating organic is not only good for you, but good for the environment. Pesticides and herbicides get into our water supply, and the water supply of wildlife. Pesticides particularly are largely responsible for killing off large colonies of bees; an insect that is detrimentally important to life on Earth. By buying organic, we're supporting a more sustainable ecosystem, and doing our part to create a healthy planet for generations to come.

I mentioned this earlier for those who wish to eat meat, that eating organic, farm-raised animals is healthier than not. It can be more expensive, but the more people who buy it, the cheaper the prices will eventually get. I'm noticing a huge drop in the prices of organic veggies these days compared to a few years ago. The biggest way we can affect change is with our pocket books.

iv.

Diet & Lifestyle Reference List

I've already talked a lot about nutrition and diet style, but in this section, I want to touch upon a few of the diet types that I think are good for someone looking to maintain perfect health. I have tried all of them and have mixed and matched the ones that work best for me. Of course these diets may or may not have disease fighting properties, and I would use them more as a maintenance part of one's lifestyle. In using food to help fix a problem, I only recommend the raw diet and/or heavy juicing.

In my humble opinion, most Asian countries have the nutrition thing down! With the exception of the types of food that over salt and over sugar, the traditional forms of Japanese, Indian, and Thai foods are very healthy.

I prefer to eat Japanese food. For all the radiation I've done, and for the sake of the stricture, I eat a lot of sushi. It makes me feel great, and does not upset my body; especially when I make it myself. I don't wonder why the people in the parts of the world that eat sushi as their main staple, have the best overall longevity.

Ayurvedic is another super healthy way to eat as it incorporates all seven flavors in each dish which creates a varied diet. If you study more about the

230

Ayurvedic lifestyle, you can learn what type of body type you have and base the foods you eat on that chart. Ayurveda hails from India.

I've changed this paragraph from the original version because the information I have about it has changed. It's not just a great "fix" diet. When doing maintenance, eating raw 90%, 50%, or even 30% of the time is going to help keep us healthy. All of us should strive for those percentages no matter what diet or lifestyle we choose.

The vegan diet is both healthy and ethical. It's very close to the perfect diet, as far as I believe, though I'm currently a pesco-vegetarian (fish eater). Most people can do very well on the vegan diet. It's a great diet to test what diet feels healthy for the individual. For those who don't know, a vegan diet allows no animal products, whatsoever. No meat, dairy, eggs, or honey.

There are several types of vegetarian diets. Vegan is one type. The ovo-vegetarian eats eggs, and the lacto-vegetarian eats dairy products, and the lacto-ovo-vegetarian eats eggs and dairy.

Pesco-vegetarian sounds like an oxy-moron, but to me it infers that yeah, the diet has fish in it, but it's primarily plant based. Sometimes I go for long periods of time without eating any fish, sometimes I need it more. Maybe other fish eaters identify more with simply being a pescetarian.

I believe fish we (as in humans) are supposed to eat fish simply because it's so healthy for us. They have beneficial oils and nutrients that are difficult, if not impossible to get from other sources. Other meats just aren't healthy, plus they're difficult to digest.

There are many other diets that can be used as healthy, like the macrobiotic diet, which I didn't use to think was appropriate enough for those of us with cancer, but since this book's first publication, I met someone who used the macrobiotic diet to keep his cancer tumors stable. When he ended the diet, the cancer began to grow again.

It's my opinion that the above listed diets coupled with a mostly gluten-free, refined sugar-free diet is the most optimum for those who want to maintain good health and/or to manage illness. Completely eliminating cow, chicken, turkey, and pig in the diet is always going to be healthier, too.

Vitamins and Supplements List

Below is a list of the vitamins I have experimented with, and/or still take. Including the companies I have come to trust, and the best places I've found to get them.

Multi-Vitamin: Vitamin Code 50 & Wiser Women/Men, by Garden of Life. The 50 & wiser has more vitamins and probiotics in them than the regular mulit-vitamin. Can find on eBay.

D3: Vitamin Code Raw D3, by Garden of Life. Can find on eBay.

Probiotics: Primal Defense Ultra, by Garden of Life. Can find on eBay.

Calcium: Red Mineral Algae, by Now. Can find on Amazon.com

Enzymes: Univase Forte, by Rocky Fork Formulas. Www.rockyforkformulas.com, or Megazyme Forte by biophix. Can be found on Amazon. If these are unavailable for some reason, there are other companies that make these particular enzymes, but it's difficult to find the ones with high enough a-chymotrypsin and trypsin. The Univase Forte has the highest I've seen with 60 mg per tablet. With the megazyme, the enzymes are less, so I just take more tablets.

Chaga: Mushroom Science is what I've taken, but any pure Chaga will do. This can be found at sunfood.com. Any TCM doctor will have this available in tea form.

Other supplements I've used in the past are milk thistle for liver health. I don't have a company I prefer for that, but I'm fairly sure Now makes a milk thistle, and I think they're a good, respectable vitamin company.

Remember that vitamins should only be taken if there is a deficiency in something, or if absorption is an issue, and then discontinued when no longer needed. A healthy, varied, diet will supply all the vitamins and minerals a body needs under normal circumstances.

Cancer Resources:
Financial/Emotional

CancerCare
Cancer
1-800-813-HOPE
Groups
www.cancercare.org
www.cancertrialshelp.org

Coalition of

Cooperative

National Patient Advocate Foundation
202-347-8009
www.npaf.org
Survivors Network

Cancer

(CSN)

Fifth Season
www.cancer.org/csn
Financial Assistance
866-459-1271
www.fifthseasonfinancial.com

Cancer.net
www.cancer.net

Colon Cancer Alliance
877-422-2030
www.ccaliance.org

chris4life
www.chris4life.org

Fight Colorectal Cancer
1-877-427-2111
www.fightcolorectalcancer.org

Sharon Osbourne
www.sharonosbourne.com/support.html

Centers for Disease Control (CDC)
http://www.cdc.gov/cancer/survivorship/uninsured.ht
m

California Department of Public Health
www.cdph.ca.gov/programs/pages/C4P/aspx

Stupid Cancer
www.stupidcancer.org/directories/money.shtml

Life Beyond Cancer Foundation
1-800-282-5223

Brenda Mehling Cancer Fund
for those between the ages of 18-40. Email for info.
info08@bmcf.net

Joe's House
For families who have to travel for treatments
1-877-563-7468

Cancer Resource Mama
www.cancerresourcemama.com

PAF/Patient Advocate Foundation
1-800-532-5274

SSI (Supplemental Security Income) is designed for people who are unable to work due to illness. It's not easy to get, even when you're very sick, so expect do so some serious hoop jumping if you go it alone.

Unless you're a stage IV at diagnosis, chances are very high you will have to go through the appeals process to get your SSI, and eventually go before a judge in a private hearing.

They made me go see one of their doctors who really didn't care what my condition was. She was basically just there to tell SSI that I was perfectly healthy. She had me bending over to touch my toes, even though it caused a lot of pain, and I could barely walk because of the not-yet-diagnosed busted tailbone. After that, I was done getting bullied, and got an attorney on it. He took care of everything, and even accompanied me to see the judge. It was all very informal. The attorney will take a portion of the back pay you're owed from SSI.

To find an SSI office near you, go to
www.ssa.gov/ssi/
Or call: 1-800-772-1213

If you need it, by all means apply for it. That's what

it's there for and what you've been paying into your entire working career. When you're well enough to work again, you'll pay into it again. The point is to get well again, and in many instances, working a stressful job isn't the way to do it; especially when you're already sick. If you're able to work a little, SSI will deduct a percentage of what you make from what they're giving you. Simply ask them or your attorney, what the SSI rules are. Actually, ask the attorney. I always get different answers from SSI on the same questions.

vii.

Alternative Treatment
Facilities & Options

Immunity Therapy Center
(Oxygen Therapy) Mexico
1-619-415-4443
1-619-407-7753
www.bioresearchinstitute.com

Oasis of Hope
(Varied Treatments) Mexico
1-619-690-8450
www.oasisofhope.com

During my research putting this part of the appendix in order, I stumbled across a website that sounded good until I saw that the doctor was claiming he had the "only" cure for cancer. Typically when I see that, I instinctively run the other way! For some reason, probably curiosity, I continued reading.

I'm amazed at the things this doctor is plugging. He's verifying many of the things I've talked about here, which surprised me. Here is his website; www.drleonardcoldwell.com.

I still believe there are many cures for cancer, but I also believe some cures kill ALL cancers. Maybe Dr. Coldwell's is one of those. I believe Dr. Gerson's is because they're primarily using diet.

Gerson Institute
1-800-443-7766
www.gerson.org

Gerson Hungarian Clinic
+36.30.6426.291

Gerson Mexico Clinic
Go to main website, and fill out application

To find a traditional Chinese medicine (TCM) doctor,
check at local hospitals if they have anyone they
recommend. That's how I found mine. There is also a
website that can help you locate one near you.
www.nccaom.org

viii.

Books, Articles, and Videos

This is a list of books for further reading. A few are articles I found online, or ones that I have used information from.

Anticancer: A New Way of Life, David Servan-Schreiber.

Buddha's Brain: The Practical Neuroscience of Happiness, Love and
                Wisdom. Rick Hanson, Richard
Mendius

The Live Food Factor: The Comprehensive Guide to the Ultimate
                Diet for Body, Mind, Spirit and
Planet. Susan
                E. Schenck, Victoria Bidwell.

Superfoods: The Food and Medicine of the Future. David Wolfe

http://www.anticancerinfo.co.uk/enzymes.html A great article on the digestive enzymes that dissolve cancer's protein barrier.

A Beautiful Truth, DVD by Garrett Kroschel.

Available on Netflix.

The Gerson Miracle, DVD by Max and Charlotte Gerson. Available on Netflix.

The following books I have not read myself, but will add here for those who want to branch out their research.

Eat Right 4 Your Type: The Individualized Diet Solution to Staying
Healthy, Living Longer, and
Achieving Your
Ideal Weight, Peter J.
D'Adamo, Catherine
Whitney.

The Book of Ayurveda: A Holistic Approach to Health and Longevity,
Judith Morrison.

Spontaneous Healing: Andrew Weil, M.D.

Spiritual Nutrition & The Rainbow Diet: Gabriel Cousens

X.
Meat Substitutes/Alternatives

Here is a list of websites, and products for meat substitutes. These are gluten-free. There are plenty of substitutes that aren't gluten-free that are very good, as well. Just use these sparingly as they are processed foods.

http://www.fakemeats.com/GlutenFreeProducts_s/43.htm

Tofu pups are sold at most grocery stores, and health food stores.

Loma Linda offers a variety of canned meat alternatives, such as hot dog alternatives that are very tasty. They can be found at Stater Bros. grocery stores usually in the tuna aisle, and at many health food stores.

xi.

Bibliography

http://www.environmentalhealthnews.org/ehs/news/wildlife-cancer.

http://martinfrost.ws/htmlfiles/chernobyl2.html.

http://npic.orst.edu/factsheets/ddtgen.pdf

http://www.rickhanson.net/writings/buddhas-brain

www.ingramcontent.com/pod-product-compliance
Lightning Source LLC
Chambersburg PA
CBHW060243290526
45789CB00001B/165